HEALTH CARE ISSUES, COSTS AND ACCESS

MEDICARE AND THE PATIENT PROTECTION AND AFFORDABLE CARE ACT

HEALTH CARE ISSUES, COSTS AND ACCESS

Additional books in this series can be found on Nova's website under the Series tab.

Additional E-books in this series can be found on Nova's website under the E-book tab.

HEALTH CARE ISSUES, COSTS AND ACCESS

MEDICARE AND THE PATIENT PROTECTION AND AFFORDABLE CARE ACT

PAUL L. SCHMIDT
EDITOR

Nova Science Publishers, Inc.
New York

For permission to use material from this book please contact us:
Telephone 631-231-7269; Fax 631-231-8175
Web Site: http://www.novapublishers.com

Library of Congress Cataloging-in-Publication Data

Medicare and the Patient Protection and Affordable Care Act / editor, Paul L. Schmidt.
p. ; cm. -- (Health care issues, costs and access)
Includes bibliographical references and index.
ISBN 978-1-61122-897-7 (hardcover : alk. paper)
1. Medicare. 2. United States. Patient Protection and Affordable Care Act. I. Schmidt, Paul L. II. Series: Health care issues, costs, and access.
[DNLM: 1. United States. Patient Protection and Affordable Care Act. 2. Medicare--legislation & jurisprudence. 3. Health Care Reform--economics--United States. 4. Health Care Reform--legislation & jurisprudence--United States. 5. Medicare--economics. WT 31]
RA412.3.M427275 2011
368.4'2600973--dc22

2010047053

Published by Nova Science Publishers, Inc. † New York

Contents

Preface

On March 30, 2010, the President signed the Health Care and Education Reconciliation Act, which modifies a number of Medicare provision in PPACA and adds several new provisions. This new and important book examines the Medicare related provisions in these Acts. Estimates from CBO and PPACA and the Reconciliation Act indicate that net reductions in Medicare direct spending will reach approximately $390 billion from 2010 to 2019.

Chapter 1- Medicare is a federal program that pays for covered health services for most persons 65 years old and older and for most permanently disabled individuals under the age of 65. The rising cost of health care, the impact of the aging baby boomer generation, and declining revenues in a weakened economy continue to challenge the program's ability to provide quality and effective health services to its 45 million beneficiaries in a financially sustainable manner.

Chapter 2- Medicare is a federal insurance program that pays for covered health care services of qualified beneficiaries. It was established in 1965 under Title XVIII of the Social Security Act as a federal entitlement program to provide health insurance to individuals 65 and older, and has been expanded over the years to include permanently disabled individuals under 65. Medicare, which consists of four parts (A-D), covers hospitalizations, physician services, prescription drugs, skilled nursing facility care, home health visits, and hospice care, among other services.

In: Medicare and the Patient Protection and Affordable Care Act ISBN: 978-1-61122-897-7
Editor: Paul L. Schmidt

Chapter 1

Medicare Provisions in the Patient Protection and Affordable Care Act (PPACA): Summary and Timeline*

Patricia A. Davis, Jim Hahn, Geoffrey J. Hoffman, Paulette C. Morgan, Julie Stone and Sibyl Tilson

Summary

Medicare is a federal program that pays for covered health services for most persons 65 years old and older and for most permanently disabled individuals under the age of 65. The rising cost of health care, the impact of the aging baby boomer generation, and declining revenues in a weakened economy continue to challenge the program's ability to provide quality and effective health services to its 45 million beneficiaries in a financially sustainable manner.

On March 23, 2010, the President signed into law H.R. 3590, the Patient Protection and Affordable Care Act (PPACA; P.L. 111-148), as passed by the Senate on December 24, 2009, and the House on March 21, 2010. The new law will, among other things, make numerous statutory changes to the Medicare program. On March 30, 2010, the President signed into law H.R. 4872, the Health Care and Education Reconciliation Act of 2010 (the "Reconciliation Act," or HCERA; P.L. 111-152), which modifies a number of Medicare provisions in PPACA and adds several new provisions.

This report, one of a series of CRS products on PPACA and the Reconciliation Act, examines the Medicare related provisions in these Acts. Estimates from CBO on PPACA and the Reconciliation Act indicate that net reductions in Medicare direct spending will reach approximately $390 billion from FY2010 to FY2019. Major savings are expected from

---

* This is an edited, reformatted and augmented version of Congressional Research Service publication, Report R41196, dated June 30, 2010.

constraining Medicare's annual payment increases for certain providers, tying maximum Medicare Advantage payments near or below spending in fee-for-service Medicare, reducing payments to hospitals that serve a large number of low-income patients, creating an Independent Payment Advisory Board to make changes in Medicare payment rates, and modifying the high-income threshold adjustment for Part B premiums. A new Hospital Insurance tax for high-wage earners will also raise approximately $87 billion over 10 years, and a new Medicare tax on net investment income, added by the Reconciliation Act, is expected to raise an additional $123 billion over 10 years.

Other provisions in PPACA address more systemic issues, such as increasing the efficiency and quality of Medicare services and strengthening program integrity. For example, PPACA requires the establishment of a national, voluntary pilot program that will bundle payments for physician, hospital, and post-acute care services with the goal of improving patient care and reducing spending. Another provision adjusts payments to hospitals for readmissions related to certain potentially preventable conditions. In addition, PPACA subjects providers and suppliers to enhanced screening before allowing them to participate in the Medicare program, and both PPACA and the Reconciliation Act increase funding for anti-fraud activities.

PPACA also improves some benefits provided to Medicare beneficiaries. For instance, Medicare prescription drug program enrollees will receive a 50% discount off the price of brand-name drugs during the coverage gap (the "doughnut hole") starting in 2011, and the coverage gap will be phased out by 2020. Other provisions expand assistance for some low-income beneficiaries enrolled in the Medicare drug program, and eliminate beneficiary copayments for certain preventive care services.

Introduction

On March 23, 2010, President Obama signed into law comprehensive health care reform legislation, the Patient Protection and Affordable Care Act (PPACA; P.L. 111-148), as passed by the Senate on December 24, 2009, and by the House of Representatives on March 21, 2010. The Act contains numerous provisions affecting Medicare payments, payment rules, covered benefits, and the delivery of care. On March 30, 2010, the President signed into law H.R. 4872, the Health Care and Education Affordability Reconciliation Act of 2010 (the Reconciliation Act, or HCERA; P.L. 111-152), as passed by both the Senate and the House on March 25, 2010. The Reconciliation Act makes changes to a number of Medicare-related provisions in PPACA and adds several new provisions.

Prior to the enactment of the health care reform legislation, CBO estimated that total mandatory annual expenditures for Medicare would grow from $501 billion in 2009 to $943 billion in 2019.[1] Cumulative spending for FY2010 to FY2019 was expected to exceed $7 trillion. CBO estimates on the Medicare-related provisions in PPACA and the Reconciliation Act indicate that absent interaction effects, net reductions in Medicare direct spending will reach approximately $390 billion over the FY2010-FY2019 period.

PPACA includes 10 titles. This report discusses selected provisions in Titles II, III, IV, V, VI, IX, and X in PPACA concerning payment and program modifications to Medicare's fee-for-service program, the Medicare Advantage (MA), and outpatient prescription drug programs; efforts to reform Medicare's payment methods; program integrity changes to address fraud, waste, and abuse; and other miscellaneous Medicare changes. Provisions that modify Medicare's graduate medical education payments to teaching hospitals, some quality measurement efforts, and other public health initiatives are not covered in this report.[2]

The Reconciliation Act includes two titles. The first title contains provisions related to health care and revenues. Subtitle B of Title I contains provisions that modify provisions in PPACA related to Medicare fee-for-service, Medicare Advantage, and Medicare outpatient prescription drug programs. Subtitle D contains provisions related to reducing waste, fraud, and abuse in Medicare. Subtitle E contains revenue related provisions including a provision that makes changes to the Medicare tax provision in PPACA. The second title includes amendments to the Higher Education Act of 1965, which authorizes most of the federal programs involving postsecondary education. This report also addresses how the Reconciliation Act changed, or added to, Medicare-related provisions in PPACA.

The body of this report begins with a discussion of the financial impact on the Medicare program by PPACA and the Reconciliation Act as estimated by CBO (the CBO score), then provides an overview of Medicare changes by provider type and program, followed by a brief discussion of the changes to address efficiencies and quality in Medicare, efforts to address long-term Medicare financing, and program integrity changes.[3] **Appendix A** provides an overview of the majority of Medicare-related provisions in PPACA and the Reconciliation Act, including a brief description of the law prior to enactment, a description of the provision, and where possible, the associated CBO score for each provision. Title X provisions of PPACA and provisions added by the Reconciliation Act are incorporated within the subject appropriate titles. Appendix B contains a timeline for provider payment update reductions including productivity adjustments (described in "Payment Rate Changes Affecting Medicare Fee-for-Service Providers"). Appendix C contains a timeline of the effective, start, or due dates of the Medicare provisions described in this report. A glossary of common acronyms used in body of the report and in the timeline appears in **Appendix D**.

Congressional Budget Office (CBO) Score

On March 20, 2010, the Congressional Budget Office (CBO) and the Joint Committee on Taxation (JCT) issued cost estimates of PPACA as amended by the Reconciliation Act.[4] Their analyses provide estimates of the direct spending and revenue effects of the combined pieces of legislation.

CBO estimates that the provisions in PPACA as amended by the Reconciliation Act that affect the Medicare, Medicaid, the State Children's Health Insurance Program (CHIP) and other federal programs will reduce direct spending by $511 billion over the FY2010-FY2019 period.[5] Medicare (absent interaction effects) accounts for approximately $390 billion of the reduction.[6] Total Medicare reductions in direct spending over the 10-year period are estimated to be about $460 billion, but these reductions are offset by Medicare payment increases of close to $70 billion.[7]

Estimates of annual Medicare spending from FY2010 through FY2019 under PPACA and the Reconciliation Act, and under prior law ("baseline") are illustrated in **Figure 1**.

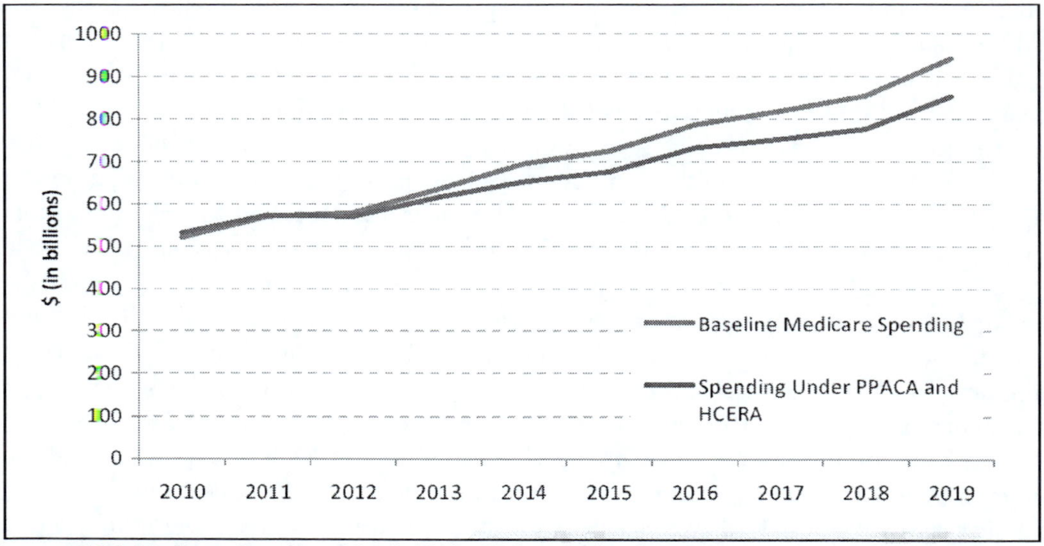

Source: CBO Medicare Baseline, March 2009; CRS analysis of CBO Cost Estimates for the PPACA as amended by the Reconciliation Act, March 20, 2010.

Figure 1. Estimates of Medicare Spending FY2010-FY2019 Prior Law and PPACA as Amended by the Reconciliation Act

As noted by CBO, the provisions that are expected to result in the largest savings include the following:

- Permanent reductions in the annual updates to Medicare's fee-for-service payment rates (other than physicians' services) will account for an estimated budgetary savings of $196.3 billion over 10 years.[8]
- Tying maximum payment rates in the Medicare Advantage program closer to spending in fee-for-service Medicare (or below that level) will account for an estimated $135 billion in savings (before interactions) over 10 years.
- Reducing Medicare payments to hospitals that serve a large number of low-income patients, known as disproportionate share (DSH) hospitals, is expected to decrease expenditures by about $22 billion.
- Modifying the high-income adjustment for Part B premiums is projected to save $25 billion over 10 years.
- Creating an Independent Payment Advisory Board to make changes in Medicare payment rates is expected to save approximately $16 billion over 10 years.

Additionally, a new Hospital Insurance tax on taxable wages over $200,000 per year for single filers ($250,000 for joint filers) is expected to raise $87 billion from FY2013 through FY2019, and a new tax on investment income is projected to raise an additional $123 billion over 10 years.

CBO estimates that Medicare spending under health care reform legislation will increase more slowly over the next 20 years compared to the past 20 years—a 6% average annual rate compared to the prior 8%.[9] CBO notes, however, that the estimates are subject to uncertainty. For example, the savings rate assumed that the sustainable growth rate (SGR) mechanism that constrains Medicare physician payment rates would go back into effect in 2010; at the time the estimate was made, physicians were facing an approximate 21% cut in payments.[10] The longer-term projections also assume that the Independent Payment Advisory Board established by PPACA will be effective in reducing costs. CBO was not able to determine whether the reduction in the growth rate would be achieved through greater efficiencies in the delivery of health care or if the payment reductions would lead to lower quality of care.[11]

Payment Rate Changes Affecting Medicare Fee-for-Service Providers

Medicare is a federal program that pays for covered health services for most persons 65 years of age and older and for most permanently disabled individuals under the age of 65. It consists of four parts, each responsible for paying for different benefits, subject to different eligibility criteria and financing mechanisms.[12] Under traditional Medicare, Part A and Part B services are typically paid on a fee-for-service basis (each service or group of services provided to a patient is reimbursed through a separate payment) using different prospective payment systems (PPS) or fee schedules.[13] Certain other services are paid on the basis of reasonable costs or reasonable charges.

In general, each year, the Centers for Medicare and Medicaid Services (CMS) issues regulations to set Medicare's payment rates to specific providers, physicians, practitioners and suppliers for the upcoming year. For instance, the program provides for annual updates of Medicare payments to reflect inflation and other factors. In some cases, these updates are linked to the consumer price index for all urban consumers (CPI-U) or to a provider-specific market basket (MB) index, which measures the change in the price of goods and services purchased by the provider to produce a unit of output. While CMS implements the payment methods through detailed rule-making, typically, the basic parameters for setting these payments, including updates over time, have been established by Congress.

In March of each year, the Medicare Payment Advisory Commission (MedPAC) makes payment update recommendations concerning Medicare's different fee-for-service payment systems to Congress.[14] To do so, MedPAC staff first examines the adequacy of the Medicare payments for efficient providers in the current year and then assesses how provider costs are likely to change in the upcoming year, including scheduled policy changes that will affect Medicare's payment rates.[15] As stated by MedPAC, Medicare's payment systems should encourage efficiency, and Medicare providers can achieve efficiency gains similar to the economy at large. This policy target links Medicare's expectations for efficiency improvements to the productivity gains achieved by firms and workers who pay taxes that fund Medicare. The amount, if any, of MedPAC's update recommendations will depend on its overall assessment of the circumstances of a given set of providers in any year. To differing extents, MedPAC's analyses and recommendations have shaped provisions in PPACA and the Reconciliation Act; that influence is noted in this report wherever applicable.

Hospitals and other Part A Providers

Part A provides coverage for inpatient hospital services, post-hospital skilled nursing facility (SNF) services, post-hospital home health services, and hospice care, subject to certain conditions and limitations. Approximately 20% of beneficiaries enrolled in Part A use these services during any year. CBO estimates that about $223 billion was spent on Part A benefits in 2008, an amount that is projected to increase to $435.2 billion in 2019. In part because of its sheer size, provisions reducing Part A spending comprise a significant proportion of the savings attributed to this legislation either through constraining payment updates or by other payment changes.

Acute Care Hospitals

Generally, the provisions of PPACA and the Reconciliation Act affecting Medicare's payments to acute care hospitals will constrain payment increases to these hospitals, restructure payments to address treatment inefficiencies, and then reshape Medicare's disproportionate share hospital (DSH) hospital subsidies. Also, the exception that permits physicians with ownership interests in a hospital to refer Medicare and Medicaid patients to that hospital will be eliminated for new physician-owned hospitals or those that did not meet certain criteria.

Specifically, PPACA will adjust Medicare's annual payment updates to Part A hospitals to account for economy-wide productivity increases for cost savings (along with certain other reductions), which is estimated to reduce Medicare spending significantly over 10 years. Under prior law, the market basket component of the physician update or the Medicare economic index (MEI) was adjusted to exclude productivity gains. The PPACA provision for adjusting payment updates for Part A hospitals will use the same measure of productivity improvement, the 10-year moving average of all-factory productivity, included in the MEI. These estimated savings include the reduction for outpatient and inpatient services for all hospitals; the savings from extending this policy to only acute care hospitals were not separately identified.[16]

Since 1986, an increasing number of acute care hospitals have received additional payments under Medicare's inpatient prospective payment system (IPPS) because they serve a disproportionate share of low-income patients. The justification for this subsidy has changed over time. Originally, the DSH adjustment was intended to compensate hospitals for their higher Medicare costs associated with the provision of services to a large proportion of low-income patients. Now, the adjustment is considered as a way to protect access to care for Medicare beneficiaries. PPACA as amended by the Reconciliation Act will reduce hospitals' DSH payments starting in FY2014 equal to 25% of what otherwise would be made, a payment that represents the empirically justified amount as determined by MedPAC in its March 2007 *Report to Congress*.[17] Acute care hospitals will be paid additional amounts, which will depend on the difference in the hospital's DSH payments under PPACA, the difference in the percentage change in the uninsured under-65 population from 2012, and the percentage of uncompensated care provided by the hospital (relative to all acute care hospitals). CBO has estimated that this policy will save $22.1 billion from FY2015 to FY2019.

Skilled Nursing Facilities (SNFs)

Medicare covers nursing home services for beneficiaries who require skilled nursing care and/or rehabilitation services following a hospitalization of at least three consecutive days. The Balanced Budget Act of 1997 (BBA 97, P.L. 105-33) required the Secretary to establish a prospective payment system (PPS) for SNF care to be phased in over three years, beginning in 1998. Under the PPS, SNFs receive a daily payment that covers all the services provided that day, including room and board, nursing, therapy, and drugs, as well as an estimate of capital-related costs. Any profits are retained by the SNF, and any losses must be absorbed by the SNF. The daily base payment is based on 1995 costs that have been increased for inflation and vary by urban or rural location. A portion of these daily payments is further adjusted for variations in area wages, using the hospital wage index, to account for geographic variation in wages. SNF per diem PPS payments are also adjusted to include a temporary 128% increase for any SNF residents who are HIV-positive or have AIDS. Section 1888(e) of the Social Security Act requires that the base payments be adjusted each year by the SNF MB update—that is, the measure of inflation of goods and services used by SNFs. In its *March 2009 Report*,[18] MedPAC found that Medicare payments to SNFs overall were adequate and recommended that the market basket update for 2010 be eliminated.

According to the CMS final rule for FY2010, published on August 11, 2009,[19] the market basket update for FY2010 is 2.2 percentage points. In addition, CMS described how it would establish a revised case-mix classification methodology (Resource Utilization Group–Version Four; RUG-IV) and implementation schedule for FY2011 (starting October 1, 2010), reflecting updated staff time measurement data derived from the recently completed Staff Time and Resource Intensity Verification (STRIVE) project, among other things. According to CMS, these revisions to the case-mix are intended to correct for changes made for FY2006, in which changes that were intended to better account for the resources used in the care of medically complex patients resulted in payments exceeding budget neutrality estimates.

The FY2010 final rule also describes changes to the RUG system for measuring and billing therapy given to Medicare SNF patients on a concurrent basis. Concurrent therapy is the practice of a professional therapist working with multiple patients at the same time, each of whom is receiving different treatments. Prior to FY2010, SNFs were allowed to bill for concurrent therapy as individual therapy time for each patient. The FY2010 final rule requires SNFs to instead calculate the therapy minutes allocated to each individual and to report only those minutes on the MDS 3.0 for billing purposes.

The FY2010 final rule also describes changes to billing for the following high-cost staff-intensive services: ventilator/respirator, tracheostomy, suctioning, IV medications, and transfusions. Prior to the implementation of the new law, the RUG billing system took into account the costs of these services when furnished within the prior 14 days, regardless of whether they were furnished prior to a patient's admission. According to CMS, the inclusion of these expenditures in the RUG billing system was intended to serve as a proxy for the higher-cost medically complex services delivered to certain categories of SNF residents. More recent analysis by CMS showed this to be a poor proxy for medical complexity. As a result, the FY2010 rule modifies this look-back period to include only services delivered after admission to a SNF.

PPACA makes four significant changes to the SNF PPS. First, starting in FY2012, all SNF market-basket annual updates will be subject to a productivity adjustment. Second, the Secretary is prohibited from implementing the revised case-mix classification methodology

(Resource Utilization Group–Version Four; RUG-IV) described in the FY2010 final rule prior to October 1, 2011. (New CMS guidance explaining the delay of the RUG-IV implementation, as a result of PPACA, has not yet been published.)[20] Third, the new law required the Secretary to implement the change specified in the FY2010 final rule to therapy that is furnished on a concurrent basis. Fourth, PPACA required the Secretary to implement the changes to the look-back period described in the FY2010 final rule to ensure that only those services furnished after admission to a SNF are used as factors in determining a SNF case mix classification.

Home Health Agencies (HHAs)

Home health agencies (HHAs) are paid under a prospective payment system (PPS), which covers skilled nursing, therapy, medical social services, aide visits, medical supplies, and other services. Durable medical equipment is not included in the home health PPS. The base payment amount for the national standardized 60-day episode rate is increased annually by an update factor that is determined, in part, by the projected increase in the home health market basket (MB) index. This index measures the changes in the costs of goods and services purchased by HHAs. HHAs are currently required to submit to the Secretary health care quality data. An HHA that does not submit the required quality data will receive an update of the MB minus two percentage points for that fiscal year.

In its *March 2009 Report*, MedPAC explained that payments to HHAs have exceeded costs by a wide margin since the PPS was implemented in 2000. Further, the continuing entry of new HHAs into Medicare, combined with adequate access to capital, suggested that HHAs were not generally at risk for becoming insolvent, and were receiving adequate, or more than adequate, payment. As a result, MedPAC recommended that the MB increase for 2010 be eliminated and that the payment coding changes scheduled by the Secretary be accelerated. Further, MedPAC recommended that HHA rates be rebased to better reflect the average costs of care.

The final rule[21] for calendar year (CY) 2010 reported that the home health (HH) MB will increase by 2.0% for that year. In addition, in an effort to address potential fraud and abuse in the use of HH outlier payments, the final rule also implemented a cap on outlier payments (i.e., payments for unusually costly 60-day episodes of care) at 10% of total payments per HHA, and no more than 2.5% of total aggregate PPS payments for all of HH.

In CY2008, CMS made refinements to the home health PPS to try to improve payment efficiencies. Specifically, the Secretary made changes to the home health agency (HHA) case-mix index to account for the relative resource utilization of different patients. These changes modified the coding or classification of different units of service that do not reflect real changes in case-mix. As a result, the national prospective 60-day episode payment rate was adjusted downward by 2.75% for CY2008, by 2.75% for each year of CY2009 and CY2010, and by 2.71% for CY2011. The final CMS rule for CY2010 maintained the 2.75% reduction to the HH PPS rates for CY2010. The final rule also required the submission of OASIS (home health patient assessment tool) data by HHAs to the Secretary as a condition for payment, and began implementing a new version of OASIS, OASIS-C January 1, 2010.

Several provisions in PPACA will impact HH payments, some of which reflect MedPAC's recommendations. For example, one provision will reduce the HH MB update by 1.0 percentage point in 2011, 2012, and 2013, and all HH MB annual updates will be subject to a productivity adjustment starting in 2015. With these changes to the market basket updates, the rate of growth in payments to HHAs will likely slow and could even fall below zero.

Another provision in PPACA requires the Secretary to rebase home health payments, starting in CY2014, by a percentage considered appropriate by the Secretary to, among other things, reflect the number, mix and level of intensity of HH services in an episode, and the average cost of providing care. Any such adjustments that would result will be required to be made before the annual payment updates are applied for that year. A four-year phase-in, ending in 2017, will be provided for, in equal increments that cannot exceed 3.5% of applicable amounts for each year.

Regarding payments, the Secretary is required to reduce the standard home health resource group (HHRG) amounts such that the aggregate reduction in payments will equal 5% of total HHA PPS payments for a period. And, similar to the CMS final rule for CY2010, the total amount of additional payments for outliers may not exceed 2.5% of the total HHA PPS payments in a given fiscal year. Also similar to the CMS final rule, starting in CY2011 the Secretary is required to establish a provider-specific annual cap of 10% of revenues that a HH agency may be reimbursed in a given year from outlier payments. For visits ending on or after April 1, 2010, and before January 1, 2016, the Secretary is directed to provide for a 3% add-on payment for HH providers serving rural areas. CMS notification on March 31, 2010, explains that CMS is currently developing instructions for the implementation of this rural add-on payment.[22]

Physicians and other Part B Providers

PPACA and the Reconciliation Act make several changes to the Medicare program that have the potential to affect physicians and how they practice in ways both small and large, immediately and over time. While some of the provisions will have clear and direct consequences, for instance by altering physician reimbursement right away, others have the potential to influence how physicians might practice in the future by changing the incentives to encourage improvements in the organization and delivery of care.

The most immediate and direct modifications include extensions of several existing demonstration programs and payment policies as well as some modifications to the Medicare fee schedule. Among the extensions of Medicare initiatives that affect physicians are the gainsharing demonstration, the extension of the work geographic index floor and revisions to the practice expense geographic adjustment under the Medicare physician fee schedule, the payment for the technical component of certain physician pathology services, and the extension of the mental health add-on to the physician fee schedule. In addition, PPACA modifies the equipment utilization factor assumption used to determine payment for advanced imaging services, creates a new demonstration project to pay for certain complex diagnostic laboratory tests, and modifies the Medicare payment for certain bone density tests.

Additional provisions have impacts for physicians that will be felt in the years to come. PPACA extends the Medicare Physician Quality and Reporting Initiative (PQRI) incentive payments through 2014 and implements an incentive (penalty) for providers who do not report quality measures beginning in 2015, while also providing for an additional bonus to physicians who meet the requirements of a continuous assessment program (the Maintenance of Certification Program, MOCP) as well as a subsequent penalty for those who do not meet the standards in the future.

PPACA requires new types of reports and data analysis under the Physician Feedback Program established under the Medicare Improvements for Patients and Providers Act of 2008 (MIPPA, P.L. 110-275) including the development of an episode grouper that combines separate but clinically related items and services into an episode of care payment for an individual, as appropriate, and the provision of reports to physicians that compare patterns of resource use of each physician to the patterns of other peer physicians. Information on Medicare physicians will be reported publicly on a new Physician Compare website to be established by CMS no later than January 1, 2011, which will eventually include information on physician performance.

PPACA also gives the Secretary (through CMS) additional flexibility to be able to review and adjust potentially misvalued codes under the physician fee schedule, establishes floors for some Medicare payments for providers who practice in states that meet the definition of a "Frontier State," and creates a new bonus payment for evaluation and management and certain general surgery services for five years beginning January 1, 2011, with the intent to expand access to primary care and general surgery services

The final category of PPACA and the Reconciliation Act provisions affecting physicians has the potential to change fundamental aspects of how physicians organize, practice, and deliver care in the future. Some of these provisions create new structures and entities, like the CMS Center for Medicare and Medicaid Innovation or the Patient-Centered Outcomes Research Institute (PCORI), while others seek to develop alternatives to traditional fee-for-service payment, such as the National Pilot Program on Payment Bundling, the shared savings program (including the accountable care organization, or ACO, model), or the value-based payment modifier under the physician fee schedule. The PCORI, combined with the efforts and experiences with the alternative payment models, could generate new information about how alternative treatments affect patient outcomes as well as evidence to support how different payment methods might alter the incentives for providers and the outcomes for patients. The Innovation Center would then have the authority and flexibility to adopt new payment alternatives, so long as certain criteria were met—for instance, maintaining quality while reducing expenditures, or improving quality without increasing expenditures. In the long run, these provisions combined have the potential to be the most substantial of the PPACA and the Reconciliation Act modifications affecting physicians and related providers. All of these changes are described in more detail in Appendix A.

Payment and Administrative Changes Affecting the Medicare Advantage Program

Medicare Advantage (MA) is an alternative way for beneficiaries to receive covered benefits. Under MA, private health plans are paid a per-person amount to provide all Medicare-covered benefits (except hospice) to beneficiaries who enroll in their plan. Payments to MA plans are determined by comparing a plan's cost of providing required Medicare benefits (bid) to the maximum amount Medicare will pay for those benefits in each area (benchmark). If a plan bid is below the benchmark, the plan is paid its bid plus a rebate equal to 75% of the difference between the bid and the benchmark. If a plan bids above the benchmark, the plan is paid the benchmark and must charge each enrollee a premium equal to the difference between the bid and the benchmark. Rebates must be used to provide benefits not covered under original Medicare. Historically, Congress has increased the benchmark amounts through statutorily specified formulas, in part, to encourage plan participation in all areas of the country. As a result, the benchmark amounts in some counties are higher than the average cost of original fee-for-service (FFS) Medicare. Benchmarks currently range from about 100% to over 150% of FFS costs.[23]

PPACA, as modified by the Reconciliation Act, changed how the maximum possible payment to MA plans is determined, in addition to other payment and administrative changes. Starting in 2012, PPACA phases in benchmarks calculated as a percentage of per capita FFS Medicare spending. County benchmarks will be set at either 95%, 100%, 107.5%, or 115% of FFS spending, with a higher percentages applied to counties with the lowest FFS spending. The phase-in will take place over two to six years. This change in the calculation of MA benchmarks would lead to *reductions* in many benchmarks.

However, PPACA *increases* benchmarks based on plan quality, with higher increases for (qualifying) quality plans in qualifying areas. Starting in 2012, plans with at least a 4-star rating on a 5-star quality rating scale will receive an increase in their benchmark. New plans or plans with low enrollment may also qualify for a benchmark increase. PPACA also varies plan rebates based on quality, with new rebates set at 50% to 70% of the difference between the plan bid and the benchmark.

In addition, PPACA requires the Secretary to apply a coding intensity adjustment to plan payments after 2010. In general, MA plan payments are risk-adjusted to account for the variation in the cost of providing care. Risk adjustment is designed to compensate plans for the increased cost of treating older and sicker beneficiaries, and thus discourage plans from preferential enrollment of healthier individuals. The Deficit Reduction Act of 2005 (P.L. 109-171, DRA) required the Secretary to adjust for patterns of diagnosis coding differences between MA plans and providers under parts A and B of Medicare for plan payments in 2008, 2009, and 2010. PPACA requires the Secretary to conduct further analyses on the differences in coding patterns and adjust for those differences after 2010. It specifies minimum coding intensity adjustments starting in 2014.

CBO estimated the provisions changing MA plan payments will save $135.6 billion over the FY2010-FY2019 period.[24] CBO also estimates that the changes will result in reduced MA enrollment and plan subsidies for extra benefits. Specifically, by 2019, estimated MA enrollment will be down by 35% (or 4.8 million) from its current 2019 estimate of 13.9 million enrollees nationwide. Average subsidies of extra benefits not covered under Medicare in 2019 are expected to decrease to an estimated $67 per month, down from a 2019-estimated amount of $135 per month. (Current average subsidies of extra benefits are approximately $87 per month).[25] The impact of payment change provisions will likely vary by geography and will depend, in part, on market competition and plan quality.

PPACA makes additional changes to the Medicare Advantage program that are expected to result in costs or savings of less than $1.0 billion over the 10-year period (2010-2019), as estimated by CBO. Each of these provisions is explained in detail in **Appendix A**.

Changes Affecting Medicare's Prescription Drug Benefit

In January 2010, the Medicare prescription drug program began its fifth year of operation. The Medicare Prescription Drug, Improvement, and Modernization Act of 2003 (MMA, P.L. 108-173) created this voluntary outpatient prescription drug benefit under a new Medicare Part D, effective January 1, 2006. At that time, Medicare replaced Medicaid as the primary source of drug coverage for beneficiaries covered under both programs (called dual eligibles). Prescription drug coverage is provided through private prescription drug plans (PDPs), which offer only prescription drug coverage, or through Medicare Advantage prescription drug plans (MA-PDs), which offer prescription drug coverage that is integrated with the health care coverage they provide to Medicare beneficiaries under Part C. Medicare's payments to plans are determined through a competitive bidding process, and enrollee premiums are tied to plan bids. Plans bear some risk for their enrollees' drug spending.

Medicare law sets out a defined standard benefit structure under the Part D benefit. In 2010, the standard benefit includes a $310 deductible and then 25% coinsurance until the enrollee reaches $2,830 in total covered drug spending. After this initial coverage limit is reached, there is a gap in coverage in which the enrollee is responsible for the full cost of the drugs (often called the doughnut hole) until total costs hit the catastrophic threshold, $6,440 in 2010. Individuals with incomes below 150% of the federal poverty level and with limited assets are eligible for the low-income subsidy (LIS). The LIS reduces beneficiaries' out-of-pocket spending by paying for all or some of the Part D monthly premium and annual deductible, and limits drug copayments to a nominal amount.

PPACA and the Reconciliation Act make several changes to the Medicare Part D program that impact beneficiary premiums and out-of-pocket costs. Specifically, PPACA increases Part D premiums for higher income enrollees; the income thresholds are to be set at the same level and in the same manner as those used to establish Part B premiums. Also, starting in 2011, consistent with a voluntary agreement with the pharmaceutical industry, Part D enrollees will be provided discounts of 50% for brand-name drugs during the coverage gap. In addition, the Reconciliation Act provides a rebate of $250 to enrollees who enter the coverage gap in 2010 and phases out the Part D doughnut hole by gradually reducing the cost-sharing during the coverage gap for both brand-name and generic drugs until it equals 25% of the negotiated price of the drug in 2020 (similar to cost-sharing under the initial coverage limit). The Reconciliation Act also reduces the rate of growth of the coverage gap from 2014 through 2019. CBO estimates that the closure of the coverage gap, taking into account the manufacturer brand-name discount, will cost $42.6 billion over 10 years.

PPACA also contains several provisions designed to improve access to and availability of LIS plans. For example, the redetermination of LIS eligibility subsequent to the death of a spouse is to be postponed for a year, and cost-sharing is eliminated for individuals receiving care under a Medicaid home and community based waiver who would otherwise require care in a medical institution or a facility. PPACA also makes changes to the methodology used to determine which plans are eligible to enroll low-income beneficiaries so that more plans could qualify and thus reduce the number of low-income beneficiaries who need to change plans from year to year. Additional funding is also provided for outreach and assistance for low-income programs. The CBO cost estimate for the changes to the low-income subsidy program in PPACA is $2.4 billion over 10 years.

PPACA also includes a number of provisions aimed at expanding consumer protections for Part D enrollees. For example, the Secretary is required to develop and maintain a centralized system to handle complaints regarding Medicare Advantage and Part D plans or their sponsors. In addition, Part D plans will be required to use a single, uniform exceptions and appeals process.

Efforts to Improve the Efficiency and Quality of Health Care Services Provided Under Medicare

By statute, Medicare is prohibited from interfering in the practice of medicine or the manner in which medical services are provided. As such, Medicare pays for virtually all covered products and services if they are determined to be medically necessary. However, there is growing evidence that some services provided to Medicare beneficiaries are not medically indicated or are unnecessary. In addition, differences in local practice patterns have resulted in substantial differences in expenditures per beneficiary across geographic areas, but with no measurable differences in health status.

In June of each year, MedPAC issues a report to Congress that examines systemic issues affecting the Medicare program and makes recommendations to increase Medicare's value, to promote its efficiency, to increase payment accuracy, and/or to realign Medicare's payment incentives.[26] For instance, MedPAC has concluded that Medicare's fee-for-service reimbursement system rewards excessive care and does not encourage service coordination or quality care. Several provisions in PPACA are consistent with MedPAC recommendations to provide adequate incentives to produce appropriate, high-quality care at an efficient price. For example, a provision in PPACA requires the establishment of a national, voluntary pilot program that will bundle payments for physician and hospital as well as post-acute care services with the goal of improving patient care and reducing spending. Another provision establishes rewards for accountable care organizations[27] that meet quality-of-care targets and reduce costs per patient relative to a spending benchmark with a share of the savings they achieve for the Medicare program. CBO estimates that this shared savings program will save Medicare $4.9 billion over FY2010-2019.

In addition, under Medicare's IPPS, acute care hospitals normally receive a full payment for patient admissions even if the readmission is preventable and related to the initial admission, the result of inadequate discharge planning at the treating hospital, or results from inadequate post-discharge care coordination. PPACA, consistent with MedPAC recommendations, adjusts payments for hospitals paid under the IPPS based on the dollar value of each hospital's percentage of potentially preventable Medicare readmissions for three conditions. The Secretary of the Department of Health and Human Services has the authority to expand the policy to include additional conditions in future years. CBO estimates that this provision will save $7.1 billion over FY2010-2019. Another provision in PPACA will also subject some hospitals to a payment penalty under Medicare for certain high-cost and common health conditions acquired in the hospital. CBO estimates that this provision will result in savings of $1.4 billion over the next 10 years.

PPACA also requires the creation of a Center for Medicare and Medicaid Innovation within CMS. The purpose of the center will be to research, develop, test, and expand innovative payment and delivery arrangements to improve the quality and reduce the cost of care provided to patients. Successful models could be expanded nationally. CBO estimates that this provision will lead to an additional savings of $1.3 billion over 10 years.

Changes to Address Medicare Sustainability

Medicare's financial operations are accounted for through two trust funds, the Hospital Insurance (HI) trust fund and the Supplementary Medical Insurance (SMI) trust fund, which are maintained by the Department of the Treasury.[28] The primary source of income credited to the HI trust fund, which finances Medicare Part A, is payroll taxes paid by employees and employers; each pays a tax of 1.45% on earnings. The trust fund is an accounting mechanism; there is no actual transfer of money into and out of the fund; rather, income to the trust fund is credited to the fund in the form of interest-bearing government securities. As long as the trust fund has a balance, the Treasury Department is authorized to make payments for it from the U.S. Treasury. The 2009 report of the Medicare Board of Trustees, however, projected that the HI trust fund would become insolvent in 2017.[29] If the HI trust fund were to become insolvent, Congress would face a decision of whether and how to ensure the continued funding of Medicare Part A, as there is currently no statutory mechanism that allows for general fund transfers to cover HI expenditures that exceed payroll tax income and trust fund account balances.

Medicare Parts B and D are financed primarily through a combination of monthly premiums paid by current enrollees and general revenues. Income from these sources is credited to the SMI trust fund.[30] Because the SMI trust fund is funded by annually adjusted premiums and general revenue transfers, it is kept in balance and does not face depletion. Growth in SMI expenditures will, however, require significant increases in beneficiary premiums and general revenue over time.

In addition to provisions that reduce annual updates to certain Medicare fee-for-service payment rates, PPACA contains several other provisions to address Medicare's financial challenges. For example, PPACA includes a provision to establish an Independent Payment Advisory Board to reduce the rate of growth in Medicare spending. Beginning in 2013, if the Chief Actuary of the Centers for Medicare & Medicaid Services (OACT) makes a determination that the projected per capita growth rate under Medicare exceeds certain spending targets in the second year following the determination, the Board is required to develop a proposal containing recommendations to reduce that per capita growth rate for submission the following year. The Board will be subject to strict fiscal and policy criteria in developing its recommendations, including limitations on the types of providers it can target between years 2015 through 2019. Recommendations made by the Board are to be implemented automatically absent congressional action. CBO estimates that this provision will save $15.5 billion between 2015 and 2019.

PPACA will also impose an additional tax of 0.9% on high-income workers with wages over $200,000 for single filers and $250,000 for joint filers effective for taxable years after December 31, 2012. The Reconciliation Act imposes a tax on unearned income, starting after

December 31, 2012. The Joint Committee on Taxation estimates that these new taxes will raise approximately $210 billion between 2013 and 2019. Another provision in PPACA freezes the income thresholds used to determine which beneficiaries are subject to higher Part B premium rates at 2010 levels through 2019. Over time, this freeze will result in a larger number of beneficiaries paying the higher premiums. CBO estimates that this provision will save the Medicare program $25 billion over 10 years. In addition, as previously noted, PPACA requires high-income Part D prescription drug program enrollees to pay higher premiums. CBO estimates that this will lead to savings of close to $11 billion over 10 years.

In an analysis of PPACA, prior to amendment by the Reconciliation Act, CBO estimated that the legislation would reduce net Part A outlays by $245 billion over FY2010-FY2019.[31] As a result of cost reductions and additional revenues raised through increased payroll taxes, CBO estimated that the HI trust fund would increase by $385 billion over the 2010-2019 period, and have a balance of about $170 billion at the end of FY2019. CBO noted, however, that the trust fund balance would still be declining, and that the HI trust fund would become insolvent a few years after 2019.[32] In a separate analysis,[33] the CMS Office of the Actuary estimates that the combination of lower Part A costs and higher tax revenues in PPACA, as amended by the Reconciliation Act, will postpone the depletion of HI trust fund assets until 2029.

CBO and the CMS Office of the Actuary both caution against combining trust fund accounting conventions with budget accounting rules. Reductions in Medicare expenditures can be used to extend the solvency of the HI trust fund *or* used to offset costs associated with expansion of health insurance coverage; using both accounting methods at the same time would result in double-counting a large share of those savings.

Changes to Address Fraud, Waste, and Abuse

Health care fraud costs the nation billions of dollars annually. Although the actual amount of money lost to fraud is unknown, the estimates range from as much as 3% of all health care expenditures to as much as 10%.[34] As health care expenditures continue to rise, developing new and innovative approaches to fight fraud in both public and private health insurance programs become increasingly important.

As the agency responsible for administering CMS conducts a variety of activities designed to prevent, detect, and investigate health care fraud. These activities are referred to as program integrity activities. CMS shares responsibility for combating health care fraud with the Department of Health and Human Services Office of the Inspector General (OIG), the Department of Justice (DOJ), and the Federal Bureau of Investigation (FBI). The OIG is an independent unit within HHS that has the primary responsibility for detecting health care fraud and abuse in federal health care programs. The FBI conducts complex fraud investigations related to both private and public health care programs, and the OIG, FBI, and CMS refer suspected cases of fraud to the DOJ for prosecution.

In general, the anti-fraud provisions contained in PPACA and the Reconciliation Act target CMS's program integrity activities, the HHS OIG and DOJ enforcement efforts, and funding for anti-fraud activities. In the area of program integrity, the legislation provides the Secretary with the authority to impose certain enhanced oversight and screening measures (i.e., licensure checks, background checks, and site visits) on providers and suppliers enrolling in Medicare, Medicaid, and CHIP. To pay for these screening measures, the legislation requires that institutional providers pay an enrollment fee. Other program integrity measures include requiring Medicare, Medicaid, and CHIP providers to implement compliance programs, providing the Secretary with enhanced authority to suspend provider payments, clarifying access to payment and claims data by law enforcement agencies, and expanding Medicare's Recovery Audit Contractor (RAC) program to Medicaid and Medicare Parts C and D.

In the area of enforcement, the legislation introduces new civil monetary penalties (CMPs) for certain types of infractions, including falsifying information on provider enrollment applications and delaying investigations and audits by the OIG. The legislation also enhances the Secretary's authority to impose penalties on MA plans for violating the terms of their contract. Practices such as enrolling individuals into new MA plans or transferring individuals from one plan to another without consent will be subject to sanctions imposed by the Secretary. Finally, PPACA increases funding for the Health Care Fraud and Abuse Control (HCFAC) program by $10 million annually for fiscal years 2011 through 2020, and the Reconciliation Act provides an additional $250 million for the period FY2011 through FY2016.

Concluding Observations

Similar to other purchasers of health care, Medicare spending has been growing much faster than the general economy, and concerns about Medicare's long-term sustainability continue to intensify. Studies by CBO, MedPAC, and others attribute most of the cost growth to the development and increasing utilization of new treatments and other forms of medical technology.

Although Medicare will have the additional challenge of higher enrollment associated with aging baby boomers, CBO estimates that most of the expected increase will result from growth in per capita costs rather than from the aging of the population.[35]

PPACA and the Reconciliation Act contain provisions designed to reduce Medicare program costs by approximately $390 billion over the next 10 years through adjustments in payments to certain types of providers, by equalizing payment rates between Medicare Advantage and fee-for-service Medicare, and by increasing efficiencies in the way that health services are paid for and delivered. There are differing views, however, about whether and to what extent Medicare savings should be used as offsets to fund the expansion of health care coverage, or whether these funds are more appropriately directed at strengthening the program's future financial standing. In addition, both CBO and the CMS Office of the Actuary caution that certain payment reductions may not be sustainable in the long term, and could possibly result in diminished quality of care and/or reduce access to needed services.[36]

Appendix A. Selected Medicare Provisions in the Patient Protection and Affordable Care Act and the Health Care and Education Reconciliation Act of 2010

This appendix provides an overview of the majority of Medicare-related provisions in PPACA and the Reconciliation Act, including a brief description of the law prior to enactment, a description of the provision and, where possible, the associated CBO score for each provision. The provisions are organized by the titles of PPACA (unless otherwise noted, the section numbers refer to PPACA provisions). Title X provisions of PPACA and Reconciliation Act provisions have been incorporated within the appropriate titles. The section number and topic of Medicare-related sections that have been omitted from this appendix are included in footnotes to the immediately preceding provision.

Title II—Role of Public Programs

Subtitle K—Protections for American Indians and Alaska Natives

Sec. 2902. Elimination of Sunset For Reimbursement for All Medicare Part B Services Furnished By Certain Indian Hospitals and Clinics. Medicare covers specified Part B services provided by, or at the direction of, a hospital or ambulatory care clinic (whether provider-based or free-standing) that is operated by the Indian Health Service (IHS) and Indian tribe (IT) or a tribal organization (TO). These services include physician services, health practitioners (physician assistants, nurse anesthetists, certified nurse-midwives, clinical social workers, clinical psychologists, and registered dietitians or nutrition professionals) and outpatient physical therapy services provided by physical or occupational therapists. Section 630 of the Medicare Prescription Drug, Improvement, and Modernization Act of 2003 (MMA, P.L. 108-173) instituted a five-year expansion of the items and services covered under Medicare Part B when furnished in, or at the direction of, IHS, IT, or TO hospitals or ambulatory care clinics, applying to items and services furnished on or after January 1, 2005. The current five-year reimbursement extension will expire on January 1, 2010. The provision amends SSA Sec. 1880(e) (1) (A) to extend the period for which IHS, IT, and TO services are reimbursed by Medicare Part B indefinitely, beginning January 1, 2010. *The CBO score is $0.1 billion for FY2010-FY2014 and is $0.2 billion for FY2010-FY2019.*

Title III—Improving the Quality and Efficiency of Health Care

Subtitle A—Transforming the Health Care Delivery System

Part I—Linking Payment to Quality Outcomes Under the Medicare Program

Sec. 3001 as modified by Sec. 10335. Hospital Value-Based Purchasing Program. Since FY2005, acute care hospitals that submit required quality data have received higher payments than those hospitals that do not submit such information under Medicare's Reporting Hospital Quality Data for Annual Payment Update (RHQDAPU) program (often referred to as the hospital pay-for-reporting program or P4P program). There are 46 quality measures collected in the RHQDAPU program that impact the FY2011 payment update. Individual hospital performance on specific quality measures and on certain conditions is available on Hospital Compare available on the CMS website. In November, 2007, CMS released a mandated report on the implementation of a Medicare hospital value-based purchasing (VBP) program, which recommends expanding the RQHDAPU program in order to financially reward hospitals differentially for performance; public reporting of performance would be a key component as well.

Under PPACA, starting for discharges on October 1, 2012, hospitals will receive value-based incentive payments from Medicare. The first year of the VBP program will be a data collection/performance year. Beginning in FY2013, hospital payments will be adjusted based on performance under the VBP program. Certain hospitals will be excluded in a fiscal year: those that are subject to payment reductions associated with reporting required quality data in that fiscal year; those that have been cited for deficiencies that pose immediate jeopardy to their patients; and those for which there are not sufficient number of measures or cases that apply to the hospital for a performance period. Acute-care hospitals in Maryland paid under their state specific Medicare system will be exempt if an annual report documents that a similar state program achieves at least comparable patient outcomes and cost savings. The Secretary is to select measures other than measures of readmissions for the hospital VBP program from those used in the RHQDAPU program. In FY2013, the measures are to cover at least five specified conditions. For discharges occurring during FY2014 and subsequently, the Secretary is to ensure that measures would include appropriate efficiency measures, such as adjusted Medicare spending per beneficiary.

The Secretary is required to establish VBP performance standards, including levels of achievement and improvement, and a methodology for assessing the total performance of each hospital. The performance standards are to be announced no later than 60 days prior to the beginning of the period. Hospitals with the highest scores will receive the largest VBP payments. There will not be a minimum performance standard in determining the performance score for any hospital. Hospitals that meet or exceed the established standards for a performance period are to receive an increased base operating diagnosis-related group (DRG) payment for each discharge in the fiscal year. Starting in FY2013, the Secretary is to fund the VBP incentive payments by reducing the base operating DRG payments for each hospital's discharges in a fiscal year by an applicable percentage. These reductions will apply to all hospitals. The applicable percentage is 1.0% in FY2013; 1.25% in FY2014; 1.5% in FY2015; 1.75% in FY2016; and 2.0% in FY2017 and in subsequent years. Certain adjustments within Medicare's inpatient hospital payment system, such as those for outliers, indirect medical education, disproportionate share hospital and low volume, will not be affected. Certain payments to sole community hospitals and Medicare dependent hospitals (for FY2012 and FY2013) will also not be affected.

Individual hospital performance on each specific quality measure, on each condition or procedure, and on total performance are all to be publicly reported. A process is to be established that allows hospitals to appeal their performance assessment and score; these appeals are to be resolved in a timely manner. There will be no judicial or administrative review of certain aspects of the VBP program. The Secretary is to consult with small rural and urban hospitals on the application of the VBP program to such hospitals. The RHAQDPU program is also to be modified. The Secretary will be able to require hospitals to submit data on measures that are not used for the determination of VBP payments. Effective for FY2013 payments, the Secretary is required to provide for appropriate risk adjustment for quality measures for outcomes of care. These measures are to be validated appropriately.

The Government Accountability Office (GAO) is required to conduct a study of the VBP program with an interim report to Congress due by October 1, 2015 and a final report due by July 1, 2017. The Secretary is also required to conduct a study of the VBP with a report to Congress due by January 1, 2016. No later than two years from enactment, three-year, budget neutral VBP demonstration projects are to be established in critical access hospitals (CAHs) and in hospitals excluded from VBP because of an insufficient volume; reports on the demonstration projects are due to Congress no later than 18 months after completion of the projects. *The CBO score is $0.0 billion for FY2010-FY2014 and is $0.0 billion for FY2010-FY2019.*

Sec. 3002 as modified by Sec. 10327. Improvements to the Physician Quality Reporting System. The Tax Relief and Health Care Act of 2006 (TRHCA, P.L. 109-432) required the establishment of a physician quality reporting system that would include an incentive payment to eligible professionals who satisfactorily report data on quality measures, based on a percentage of the allowed Medicare charges for all such covered professional services. CMS named this program the Physician Quality Reporting Initiative (PQRI). The Medicare Improvements for Patients and Providers Act of 2008 (MIPPA, P.L. 110-275) made this program permanent and extended the bonuses through 2010; the incentive payment was increased from 1.5% of total allowable charges under the physician fee schedule in 2007 and 2008 to 2% in 2009 and 2010.

PPACA extends PQRI incentive payments through 2014 and implements an incentive (penalty) for providers who do not report quality measures beginning in 2015. Eligible professionals who successfully report in 2010 are to receive a 1% bonus in 2011; those who successfully report in 2011, 2012, and 2013 will receive a 0.5% bonus in 2012, 2013, and 2014, respectively.

An additional 0.5% incentive payment will be available in years 2011 through 2014 for eligible professionals who also meet the requirements of a Maintenance of Certification Program (MOCP), defined as a continuous assessment program that "advances quality and lifelong learning and self-assessment of board certified specialty physicians" by focusing on the competencies of patient care, medical knowledge, practice-based learning, interpersonal and communication skills and professionalism. MOCPs will require the physician to (1) maintain a valid, unrestricted medical license in the United States, (2) participate in educational and self-assessment programs that require an assessment of what was learned, (3) demonstrate, through a formalized, secure examination, that the physician has the fundamental diagnostic skills, medical knowledge, and clinical judgment to provide quality care in their respective specialty, and (4) successfully complete the MOCP practice assessment.

These eligible professionals will be required to participate in and successfully complete a qualified MOCP practice assessment more frequently than is required to qualify for or maintain board certification status. The MOCP is to submit information to the Secretary on behalf of the eligible professional that the professional has successfully met the program criteria and on the survey of patient experience with care, if requested. The provision authorizes the Secretary to incorporate participation and successful completion in a MCOP into the composite of measure of quality of care furnished pursuant to the physician fee schedule payment modifier.

Subsequently, eligible professionals who failed to participate successfully in the program would face a 1.5% payment penalty in 2015, and a 2% payment penalty in 2016 and in subsequent years. The incentive payments and adjustments in payment will be based on the allowed charges for all covered services furnished by the eligible professional, based on the applicable percentage of the fee schedule amount. The provision also requires CMS to develop a plan to integrate the PQRI program with the standards for meaningful use of certified electronic health records as created in the American Recovery and Reinvestment Act of 2009. *CBO estimates that the provision would cost $600 million over FY2010-FY2014 and $300 million over FY2010-2019; savings will accrue beginning in 2016 and in subsequent years.*

Sec. 3003. Improvements to the Physician Feedback Program. MedPAC, GAO and others have recently recommended providing information to physicians on their resource use. MedPAC asserts that physicians would be able to assess their practice styles, evaluate whether they tend to use more resources than their peers or what evidence-based research (if available) recommends, and revise practice styles as appropriate. MedPAC notes that in certain instances, the private sector use of feedback has led to a small downward trend in resource use. The GAO noted that certain public and private health care purchasers routinely evaluate physicians in their networks using measures of efficiency and other factors and that the purchasers it studied linked their evaluation results to a range of incentives to encourage efficiency.

MIPPA established a physician feedback program with the intent to improve efficiency and to control costs. Under the Physician Feedback Program, the Secretary will use Medicare claims data to provide confidential reports to physicians that measure the resources involved in furnishing care to Medicare beneficiaries. The resources to be considered in this program may be measured on an episode basis, on a per capita basis, or on both an episode and a per capita basis. The GAO will conduct a study of the Physician Feedback Program, including the implementation of the Program, and will submit a report to Congress by March 1, 2011, containing the results of the study, together with recommendations for such legislation and administrative action as the Comptroller General determines appropriate.

This PPACA provision requires new types of reports and data analysis under the Physician Feedback Program. Not later than January 1, 2012, the Secretary is to develop an episode grouper that combines separate but clinically related items and services into an episode of care for an individual, as appropriate. Beginning with 2012, the Secretary will also be required to provide reports to physicians that compare patterns of resource use of the individual physician to such patterns of other physicians.

In preparing these reports, the Secretary is to establish methodologies as appropriate to (i) attribute episodes of care, in whole or in part, to physicians, (ii) identify appropriate physicians for purposes of comparison, and (iii) aggregate episodes of care attributed to a physician into a composite measure per individual. In preparing these reports, the Secretary is required to make appropriate adjustments, including adjustments (i) to account for differences in socioeconomic and demographic characteristics, ethnicity, and health status of individuals, and (ii) to eliminate the effect of geographic adjustments in payment rates. *CBO estimates that this provision will have no effect on spending over the 5-year or 10-year budget window.*

Sec. 3004. Quality Reporting for Long-term Care Hospitals, Inpatient Rehabilitation Hospitals and Hospice Programs. Under current law, inpatient rehabilitation facilities (IRFs), long term care hospitals (LTCHs) and hospices are not required to report quality data to the Centers for Medicare and Medicaid Services (CMS). Medicare pays for inpatient care provided by IRFs and LTCHs, and for hospices, using different prospective payment systems (PPS). Each PPS is updated annually using a market basket (MB) index which measures the estimated change in the price of goods and services purchased by the provider to produce a unit of output. Under this provision of PPACA, the Secretary is directed to establish quality reporting programs for LTCHs, IRFs, and hospices. Starting in rate year (RY) 2014, LTCHs will be required to submit data on specified quality measures. This requirement will start in FY2014 for IRFs and hospices. Entities that do not comply will have a reduction in their annual update of 2 percentage points. The reduction could result in an annual update that is less than 0.0 which would result in a basis of payment that is lower than in the preceding year. Any reduction is not to affect payments in subsequent years. The required measures affecting these payments are to be published no later than October 1, 2012. The providers will be able to review the data prior to being publically available. *The CBO score is $0 for FY2010-FY2014 and -$0.1 billion for FY2010-FY2019.*

Sec. 3005. Quality Reporting for PPS-Exempt Cancer Hospitals. Eleven cancer hospitals are exempt from the Medicare inpatient prospective payment system (IPPS) used to pay inpatient hospital services provided by acute care hospitals. As part of these exemptions, these facilities are paid on a reasonable cost basis for providing inpatient services, subject to certain payment limitations and incentives. Currently, there are no quality reporting requirements for these hospitals. Under this provision, the Secretary is directed to establish quality reporting programs for IPPS-exempt cancer hospitals starting FY2014. These measures are to be published no later than October 1, 2012. The providers will be able to review the data prior to being publically available. *The CBO score is $0.0 billion for FY2010-FY2014 and $0.0 billion for FY2010-FY2019*

Sec. 3006 as modified by Sec. 10301. Plans for a Value-Based Purchasing Program for Skilled Nursing Facilities (SNFs), Home Health Agencies (HHAs), and Ambulatory Surgical Centers (ASCs). Under this provision, the Secretary of the Department of Health and Human Services (HHS) is required to develop three plans (for HHAs, SNFs, and ASCs) to implement Medicare value-based purchasing programs and submit them to Congress no later than January 1, 2011, for ASCs, and no later than October 1, 2011, for HHAs and SNFs. These plans are required to consider the following: (1) the ongoing development, selection, and modification process of measures, to the extent feasible and practicable, of all dimensions of quality and efficiency; (2) the reporting, collection, and validation of quality data; (3) the structure of value-based payment adjustments, including the determination of thresholds or improvements in quality that would substantiate a payment adjustment; (4) methods for the public disclosure of information on performance; and (5) other issues determined appropriate by the Secretary. In developing this plan, the Secretary is required to consult with relevant affected parties and consider experience with such demonstrations that the Secretary determines are relevant to the value-based purchasing program. *The CBO score is $0.0 billion for FY2010-FY2014 and $0.0 billion for FY2010-FY2019.*

Sec. 3007. Value-Based Payment Modifier Under the Physician Fee Schedule. Under this provision, the Secretary of HHS is required to establish and apply a separate, budget-neutral payment modifier to the Medicare physician fee schedule. The separate payment modifier is to be based on the relative quality and cost of the care provided by physicians or physician groups. Quality of care is to be evaluated on a composite of risk-adjusted measures of quality established by the Secretary, such as measures that reflect health outcomes. Costs, defined as expenditures per individual, are to be evaluated based on a composite of appropriate measures of costs established by the Secretary that eliminate the effect of geographic adjustments in payment rates and take into account risk factors (such as socioeconomic and demographic characteristics, ethnicity, and health status of individuals) and other factors determined appropriate by the Secretary.

By January 1, 2012, the Secretary is required to publish the specific measures of quality and cost, the specific dates for implementation of the payment adjustment, and the proposed prospective performance period. The Secretary is to begin implementing the value-based payment adjustment in the 2013 rulemaking process. During the performance period, which begins in 2014, the Secretary is to provide information to physicians about the value of care they provide, as reflected by the measures of relative quality and cost. The Secretary will be required to apply the payment modifier for items and services furnished beginning on January 1, 2015, for specific physicians and groups of physicians the Secretary determines appropriate, and not later than January 1, 2017, for all physicians and groups of physicians. The Secretary is to apply the payment modifier in a manner that promotes systems-based care and takes into account the special circumstances of physicians or groups of physicians in rural areas and other underserved communities. *CBO estimates that this provision will have no effect on spending over the 5-year or 10-year budget window.*

Sec. 3008. Payment Adjustment for Conditions Acquired in Hospitals. Medicare pays acute care hospitals using the inpatient prospective payment system (IPPS), where each patient is classified into a Medicare severity adjusted diagnosis-related group (MS-DRG). Generally, except for outlier cases, a hospital receives a predetermined amount for a given MS-DRG regardless of the services provided to a patient. In some instances, Medicare patients may be assigned to a different MS-DRG with a higher payment rate based on secondary diagnoses. Starting October 1, 2008, hospitals did not receive additional Medicare payment for complications that were acquired during a patient's hospital stay for certain select conditions. These hospital acquired conditions (HACs) are: (1) high cost, high volume, or both; (2) identified though a secondary diagnosis that will result in the assignment to a different, higher paid MS-DRG; and (3) reasonably preventable through the application of evidence-based guidelines. Under this provision, starting for discharges during FY2015, acute care hospitals in the top quartile of national, risk-adjusted hospital acquired condition (HAC) rates for an applicable period in a fiscal year are to receive 99% of their otherwise applicable payment.[37] Acute care hospitals in Maryland paid under their state specific Medicare system will be exempt if an annual report documents that a similar state program achieves at least comparable quality outcomes and cost savings. Prior to FY2015, the hospitals are tol receive confidential reports with respect to their HAC conditions which will be made publicly available on the Hospital Compare Internet website after the hospital has the opportunity to review and correct the data. There will be no administrative or judicial review of certain aspects of the program. The Secretary is required to submit a report to Congress by January 1, 2012, with recommendations with respect to expanding Medicare's HAC payment policy to other facilities, including IRFs, LTCHs, hospital outpatient departments, inpatient psychiatric facilities, cancer hospitals, skilled nursing facilities, ambulatory surgery centers and health clinics. *The CBO score is $0.0 billion for FY2010-FY2014 and -$1.4 billion for FY2010-FY2019.*

Sec. 10322 Quality Reporting for Psychiatric Hospitals. Under current law, psychiatric hospitals are not required to report quality data to CMS. Medicare pays for inpatient care provided by inpatient psychiatric facilities (IPFs) using a unique prospective payment system (PPS) with annual payment increases based on a market basket (MB) index which measures the estimated change in the price of goods and services purchased by the provider to produce a unit of output. Under this provision, the Secretary is directed to establish quality reporting programs for IPFs starting in rate year 2014 (July 1, 2013). Entities that do not comply will have a reduction in their annual update of 2 percentage points. The reduction could result in an annual update that is less than 0.0 which would lower payments from the preceding year. Any reduction is not applied to payments in subsequent years. The measures will be endorsed by a consensus organization under contract to develop quality measures to the extent practicable and feasible; unendorsed measures may be adopted if endorsed measures have been considered. The required measures affecting these payments are to be published no later than October 1, 2012. The providers will be able to review the data prior to being publically available. The quality data will be published on the Internet website of CMS. *CBO did not separately score this provision.*

Sec. 10326. Pilot Testing Pay-For-Performance Programs for Certain Medicare Providers. Under this provision, no later than January 1, 2016, a pilot pay-for-performance program is to be established for IPFs, LTCHs, IRFs, IPPS-exempt cancer hospitals, and hospice programs. Medicare requirements and those in Title XI and Title XVIII of the SSA are to be waived as necessary. Payments under this section for each provider type will be established so that spending will not be increased. The Secretary will be able to expand the duration and scope of the pilot project at any point after January 1, 2018, if the Secretary determines that such expansion would reduce Medicare spending without reducing quality of care or improve the quality of care and reduce spending. The Chief Actuary of CMS is to certify that an expansion would reduce Medicare spending. Finally, the Secretary is required to determine that an expansion would not deny or limit the coverage or provision of Medicare benefits. *The CBO score is $0.0 billion for FY2010-FY2014 and $0.0 billion for FY2010-FY2019.*

Sec. 10331. Public Reporting of Performance Information. SSA §1848(m)(5)(G) requires the Secretary to post on the CMS Internet website a list of eligible professionals who satisfactorily submitted data on quality measures as part of the Physician Quality Reporting Initiative (PQRI). In addition, Sec. 131(d) of the Medicare Improvements for Patients and Providers Act of 2008 requires the Secretary to develop a plan to transition to a value-based purchasing program for payment under the Medicare program for covered professional services. Not later than May 1, 2010, the Secretary is required to submit a report to Congress containing the plan and recommendations for legislative and administrative action.

This section of PPACA requires the Secretary, not later than January 1, 2011, to develop a Physician Compare Internet website with information on physicians enrolled in the Medicare program. In addition, the Secretary is required, not later than January 1, 2013, to implement a plan for making publicly available information on physician performance through Physician Compare. The section requires the Secretary to, in developing and implementing this plan, include (1) processes to assure that data made public is statistically valid and reliable; (2) processes by which providers whose performance is being publicly reported to have an opportunity to review individual results prior to publication; (3) processes to assure that the implementation of the plan provide a robust and accurate portrayal of a physician's performance; (4) data that reflects the care provided to all patients seen by physicians to the extent such information would provide a more accurate portrayal of physician performance; (5) processes to ensure appropriate attribution of care; (6) processes to ensure timely statistical performance feedback is provided to physicians; and (7) implementation of computer and data systems by CMS that support valid, reliable and accurate public reporting activities authorized under this section. The section also requires the Secretary, in developing the plan under this section, to consider the plan to transition to a value-based purchasing program for physicians and other practitioners developed under Sec. 131 of MIPPA. The Secretary is required to submit to Congress a report on the Physician Compare Internet website, including information on the plans to collect and publish data on physician quality and efficiency. Finally, the Secretary will be allowed to establish a demonstration program to provide financial incentives to Medicare beneficiaries who are furnished services by high quality physicians. *The CBO score is $0.0 billion for FY2010-FY2014 and $0.0 billion for FY2010-FY2019.* [38]

Part III—Encouraging Development of New Patient Care Models

Sec. 3021 as modified by Sec. 10306. Establishment of Center for Medicare and Medicaid Innovation Within CMS. The Social Security Amendments of 1967, as amended by the Social Security Amendments of 1972, provide the Secretary with broad authority to develop and engage in experiments and demonstrations to test new approaches to paying providers, delivering health care services, or providing benefits to beneficiaries participating in federal health care programs. All demonstrations are required to be budget neutral and be approved by the Office of Management and Budget (OMB) prior to implementation.

Scope. This provision requires the Secretary, no later than January 1, 2011, to establish a Center for Medicare and Medicaid Innovation (CMI) within CMS. The purpose of the CMI is to test innovative payment and service delivery models to reduce program expenditures under Medicare, Medicaid, and CHIP while preserving or enhancing the quality of care furnished to individuals under such titles. In selecting these models, the Secretary is also required to give preference to models that improve the coordination, quality, and efficiency of health care services. In carrying out its functions, the Secretary is required to consult with relevant federal agencies and experts in medicine and health care management.

Testing (Phase I). The Secretary is required to select models that address a defined population with poor clinical outcomes or avoidable expenditures. The provision provides the

Secretary with the authority to limit testing to certain geographic areas and select demonstration models that address a variety of themes, including medical homes, coordinated care, alternative payment mechanisms, HIT, medication management, patient education, integrated care for dual-eligibles, care for cancer patients, post-acute care, chronic care management, telehealth, and collaboration among mixed provider types. The Secretary will not have to require, as a condition for testing, that the model be budget neutral initially with respect to expenditures. When selecting models, the Secretary is authorized to consider additional factors such as whether the model includes a process for managing patient care plans, places the applicable individual at the center of the care team, utilizes technology, and demonstrates effective linkage with other private and public sector payers, among other elements.

Evaluation. The Secretary is required to conduct an evaluation of each model tested and make the evaluations publicly available in a timely fashion. Evaluations are required to include an analysis of (1) the quality of care furnished under the model, including the measurement of patient-level outcomes and patient-centeredness criteria as determined by the Secretary, and (2) the changes in spending. The Secretary may require States and other entities participating in the demonstrations to collect and report information necessary to evaluate these models.

Termination Authority. The provision requires the Secretary to terminate or modify demonstrations that do not meet one of three conditions: (1) improve quality without increasing spending; (2) reduce spending without reducing quality; or (3) improve quality and reduce spending.

Expansion Authority (Phase II). Taking into account the results of an evaluation, the Secretary has the authority to expand the duration and scope of a demonstration, including nationwide, if the Secretary determines that an expansion would: (1) reduce spending without reducing quality or improve quality without increasing spending; (2) the CMS Office of the Actuary certifies that an expansion would reduce (or not increase) net program spending under applicable titles; and (3) not deny or limit coverage.

Waiver Authority. The provision grants the Secretary the authority to waive requirements of Titles XI, Titles XVIII, and sections 1902(a)(1), 1902(a)(13), and 1902(m)(2)(A)(iii) as necessary to conduct these demonstrations. The provision also exempts the testing, evaluation, and expansion of demonstrations from Chapter 35 of title 44, the Paperwork Reduction Act (PRA), which requires federal agencies to receive OMB approval for each collection of information request.

Funding. The provision appropriates $5 million for the design, implementation, and evaluation of models for FY2010; $10 billion for the activities under this section for the years 2011 through 2019; and $10 billion for the activities initiated under this section for each subsequent 10-year fiscal period beginning with 2020. Amounts are available until expended. The provision requires that no less than $25 million be allocated to design, implement, and evaluate the specific models identified in this provision.

Oversight. Beginning in 2012, the Secretary is required to submit to Congress, at least once every other year, a report on the activities performed by the CMI. Reports are required to include a description of the demonstrations, the number of participants, the amount of payments made on behalf of these participants, models chosen for expansion, and evaluation results. Reports are also required to include recommendations for legislative action to facilitate the development and expansion of such models nationwide. *The CBO score is $0.7 billion for FY2010-FY2014 and -$1.3 billion for FY2010-FY2019.*

Sec. 3022 as modified by Sec. 10307. Medicare Shared Savings Program. In April 2005, CMS initiated the Physician Group Practice (PGP) demonstration, which offers 10 large practices the opportunity to earn performance payments for improving the quality and cost-efficiency of health care delivered to Medicare fee-for-service beneficiaries. Accountable care organizations (ACOs) would go beyond the PGP model, which is based on physician groups, to include additional providers.

The provision allows groups of providers who voluntarily meet certain statutory criteria, including quality measurements, to be recognized as ACOs and be eligible to share in the cost-savings they achieve for the Medicare program. Beginning no later than Jan. 1, 2012, this shared savings program will enable eligible ACOs to qualify for an annual incentive bonus if they achieve a threshold savings amount, established by the Secretary, for total per beneficiary spending under Medicare Parts A and B for those beneficiaries assigned to the ACO. An eligible ACO is defined as a group of providers and suppliers who have an established mechanism for joint decision making, and are required to participate in the shared savings program for a minimum of three years, among other requirements. An ACO includes practitioners (physicians, regardless of specialty; nurse practitioners; physician assistants; and clinical nurse specialists) in group practice arrangements; networks of practices; and partnerships or joint-venture arrangements between hospitals and practitioners, among others.

In each year of the three-year agreement period, an ACO will be eligible for a shared savings payment only if the estimated average per capita Medicare expenditures for Parts A and B services, adjusted for beneficiary characteristics is at least the specified percentage below the applicable benchmark. This appropriate percentage is to account for the normal variation in expenditures based on the number of beneficiaries assigned to the ACO. The ACO's benchmark for each agreement period is to be based on the most recent available three years of per beneficiary Part A and B spending for its assigned beneficiaries. This benchmark will be adjusted for beneficiary characteristics and updated by the projected absolute growth in national per capital expenditures for Part A and B FFS Medicare services, as estimated by the Secretary. The benchmark will be reset at the start of each agreement period. Subject to attaining quality performance standards, an ACO will receive a percentage of the difference between the estimated average per capita Medicare expenditures in a year, adjusted for beneficiary characteristics, under the ACO and the ACO's benchmark. The remainder of the difference will be retained by the program. The Secretary is to establish limits on the total amount of shared savings that may be paid to an ACO.

The Secretary may use a partial capitation model or other payment models. Under the partial capitation model, a qualifying ACO would be at financial risk for some, but not all, of the Part A and B items and services. The Secretary may limit participation in this model in highly integrated systems capable of bearing risk. Also, spending under this model cannot result in greater spending than would otherwise be expended if the model were not implemented.

To earn the incentive payment, the organization is to submit data pertaining to quality and fulfill certain quality requirements related to clinical processes and outcomes, patient and caregiver experience of care, and utilization measures. The Secretary has the authority to adjust the savings thresholds to account for the varying sizes of participating ACOs. If the Secretary determines that an ACO has taken steps to avoid at-risk patients in order to reduce the likelihood of increasing costs, the Secretary is authorized to impose an appropriate sanction, including terminating agreements with participating ACOs. *The CBO score is -$0.5 billion for FY2010-FY2014 and -$4.9 billion for FY2010-FY2019.*

Sec. 3023 as modified by Sec. 10308. National Pilot Program on Payment Bundling. As Medicare beneficiaries with complex health conditions and multiple co-morbidities move between hospital stays and a range of post-acute care providers, Medicare makes separate payments to each provider for covered services. The Medicare Payment Advisory Commission (MedPAC), among others, has suggested that Medicare test new incentives and payment models to encourage providers to better coordinate across patients' episodes of care and to evaluate the full spectrum of care a patient may receive during these episodes.

Under this provision, no later than January 1, 2013, the Secretary is required to establish, test and evaluate alternative payment methodologies for Medicare services through a five-year, national, voluntary pilot program. This program is to be designed to provide incentives for providers to coordinate patient care across the continuum and to be jointly accountable for an entire episode of care around a hospitalization. An episode of care is the full period that a patient stays in a hospital plus the first 30 days following discharge. The Secretary will be able to expand the duration and scope of the pilot after January 1, 2016, if the Secretary, with certification from the Chief Actuary of CMS, determines that such expansion would reduce Medicare spending without reducing quality of care, among other things.

The Secretary is required to develop provider payment methods that could include bundled payments and bids from entities for episodes of care. The bundled payment is to comprehensively cover the costs of applicable services, and other appropriate services, including acute care inpatient services; physicians' services delivered in and outside of an acute care hospital setting; outpatient hospital services including emergency department services; post-acute care services, including HH services, skilled nursing services, inpatient rehabilitation services; inpatient hospital services furnished by a LTCH; among others. Participating beneficiaries are to be entitled, to or enrolled in, Medicare Part A and enrolled for benefits under Medicare Part B. Beneficiaries cannot be enrolled in Medicare Advantage or a Program for All-Inclusive Care for the Elderly (PACE). Beneficiaries can have one or more of 10 conditions selected by the Secretary.

The payment methodology is also to include payment for services, such as care coordination, medication reconciliation, discharge planning and transitional care services, and other patient-centered activities, as determined appropriate by the Secretary. Payments for items and services cannot result in spending more than would otherwise be expended for such entities if the pilot program were not implemented. No later than three years after implementation, the Secretary is required to submit to Congress a final evaluation of this program. *The CBO score is $0.0 billion for FY2010-FY2014 and $0.0 billion for FY2010-FY2019.*

Sec. 3024. Independence at Home Demonstration Program. The Secretary is required to conduct a Medicare demonstration program, beginning no later than January 1, 2012, to test a payment incentive and service delivery model that uses physician- and nurse practitioner-directed home-based primary care teams designed to reduce expenditures and improve health outcomes in the provision of items and services to certain chronically ill Medicare beneficiaries. The Secretary is to enter into agreements with qualifying independence at home medical practices, legal entities comprised of an individual physician or nurse practitioner or group of physicians and nurse practitioners that provide care as part of a team that includes physicians, nurses, physician assistants, pharmacists, and other health and social services staff, as appropriate. These practice staff are to have experience providing home-based primary care services to applicable beneficiaries. Practice staff are also required to make in-home visits, and be available 24 hours per day, 7 days per week to implement care plans tailored to the individual beneficiary's chronic conditions and designed to reduce expenditures and improve health outcomes in the provision of items and services to applicable beneficiaries.

The Secretary is required to establish a methodology for sharing savings with independence at home medical practices that have expenditures below an annual target spending level. The annual spending target (established by the Secretary) will be the amount the Secretary estimates would have been spent in the absence of the demonstration, for items and services covered under Medicare parts A and B provided to applicable beneficiaries. Subject to performance on quality measures, qualifying practices will be eligible to receive incentive payments if actual annual expenditures for applicable beneficiaries are less than the estimated spending target. Incentive payments are to be equal to a portion (as determined by the Secretary) of the amount by which actual expenditures (including incentive payments) are estimated to be less than 5% less than the estimated annual spending target.

Agreements with practices under the program cannot cover more than a three-year period. The Secretary is required to conduct an independent evaluation of the demonstration and submit to Congress a final report on the demonstration's best practices and the impact of the pilot program on coordination of care, expenditures under this provision, access to services, and the quality of health care services provided to applicable beneficiaries. The Secretary will also be required to submit a plan, no later than January 1, 2016, for expanding the program if the Secretary determines that such expansion would result in improving or not reducing the quality of patient care and reducing spending under this provision. The provision appropriates to the CMS Program Management Account $5 million for each of fiscal years 2010 through 2015 to administer the demonstration program. *The CBO score is $0.0 billion for FY2010-FY2014 and $0.0 billion for FY2010-FY2019.*

Sec. 3025 as modified by Sec. 10309. Hospital Readmissions Reduction Program. Medicare pays for inpatient care provided by acute care hospitals using an inpatient prospective payment system (IPPS) where each patient is assigned to a MS-DRG and paid based on an estimate of the average resources needed to care for a patient with specific diagnoses. Certain atypical cases may qualify for additional outlier payments. Certain hospitals receive additional indirect medical education (IME) payments because of their status as a teaching hospital, because they qualify for disproportionate share hospital (DSH) payments or because they treat a small number (or low volume) of Medicare patients. Certain types of hospitals that qualify as sole community hospitals (SCHs) or Medicare dependent hospitals (MDHs) receive additional hospital specific payments. Medicare pays for inpatient services provided by acute care hospitals in Maryland using a state specific reimbursement system established under a waiver. Medicare pays for inpatient services in other types of hospitals such as inpatient rehabilitation facilities (IRFs), inpatient psychiatric facilities (IPFs), children's hospitals, and long-term care hospitals using different reimbursement systems.

According to Medicare Payment Advisory Commission's (MedPAC), in 2005, 6.2% of acute care hospitalizations of Medicare beneficiaries resulted in readmission within 7 days and 17.6% of hospitalizations resulted in readmission within 30 days. The 17.6% of hospital readmission accounted for $15 billion in Medicare spending.

Under this provision, starting for discharges on October 1, 2012, the Secretary is to establish a hospital readmissions reduction program for certain potentially preventable Medicare inpatient hospital readmissions covering 3 conditions with high volume or high rate (or both). Medicare's base operating DRG payment amounts will be reduced by an adjustment factor. Certain components of Medicare hospital payments will be exempt from these payment reductions, including outlier, IME, DSH, and low volume payments. Hospital specific payments made to SCHs and MDHs will be exempt in FY2012 and FY2013 as well. Acute care hospitals in Maryland will be exempt from these payment adjustments if a comparable state program achieves the same or higher patient outcomes and cost savings.

The adjustment factor for a hospital in a fiscal year is to be the greater of (1) a floor adjustment factor equal to a reduced percentage of the discharge payment or (2) the excess readmissions ratio for the applicable fiscal year. The floor adjustment factor will be 0.99 of the discharge payments in FY2013, 0.98 of the discharge in FY2014, 0.97 in FY2015 and in subsequent fiscal years. The excess readmissions ratio is to equal 1 minus the ratio of the aggregate payments for excess readmissions for the hospital divided by the aggregate payments for all discharges. (Each component of this formula is specified in the provision.) Excess readmissions includes readmissions over an established minimum number for the specific applicable condition within a certain period for a hospital.

An applicable condition is defined as a condition or procedure that represents high volume (above a minimum threshold) or high expenditures for Medicare or meets other specified criteria that also satisfies certain measures of readmissions (that have been endorsed by a consensus-based entity with a performance measurement contract under Section 1890 of the Social Security Act). Readmissions do not include those readmissions that are unrelated to the prior discharge, such as a planned readmission or a transfer to another hospital. Beginning in FY2015, the number of applicable conditions are to be expanded beyond the initial 3 conditions to 4 additional conditions that were identified by MedPAC in its June, 2007, *Report to Congress* and other appropriate conditions. These additional conditions do not necessarily need to be endorsed by a consensus based organization as long as due consideration has been given to such endorsed or adopted measures.

Readmission information for acute care hospitals is to be made publically available after a hospital has the opportunity to review and correct the data prior to being made public. No judicial and administrative review will be permitted for certain aspects of the readmission program. Readmission data for all patients is to be submitted by acute care hospitals, IRFs, IPFs, children's hospitals, and LTCHs and be made publically available after appropriate review. The required data is to be able to be submitted by a state or other appropriate entity rather than by each hospital.

No later than two years after enactment, a program to improve readmission rates through the use of patient safety organizations is to be established for eligible hospitals. Eligible hospitals are those with historically high rates of risk adjusted readmissions that have not taken appropriate steps to reduce readmissions and improve patient safety. Eligible hospitals and patient safety organizations will be required to report on the processes used to improve readmission rates and resulting impact on such readmissions. *The CBO score is -$0.5 billion for FY2010-FY2014 and -$7.1 billion for FY2010-FY2019.*

Sec. 3026. Community-Based Care Transitions Program. The provision establishes a five-year Community Care Transitions Program under Medicare beginning January 1, 2011. Under this program, the Secretary is to fund eligible hospitals (with high admission rates, as defined under section 3025 of this bill) and certain community-based organizations (that provide transition services across a continuum of care through arrangements with certain hospitals and whose governing body includes sufficient representation of multiple health care stakeholders) that furnish improved care transition services to high-risk Medicare beneficiaries. High-risk Medicare beneficiaries refer to beneficiaries who have attained a minimum hierarchical condition category score, as determined by the Secretary, based on a diagnosis of multiple chronic conditions or other risk factors associated with a hospital readmission or substandard transition into post-hospitalizations. Such diagnoses or risk factors could include cognitive impairment, depression, or a history of multiple readmissions.

Applications by community-based organizations and hospitals to participate in this program will be required to propose at least one care transition intervention, other than discharge planning, such as initiating care transition services for targeted high-risk beneficiaries no later than 24 hours prior to the hospital discharge; arranging timely post-discharge follow-up to educate patients and, as appropriate, the primary caregiver, about responding to health symptoms that may indicate additional health problems or a deteriorating condition; among others. In selecting participating entities, the Secretary will be required to prioritize those entities that participate in a program administered by the Administration on Aging or provide services to medically underserved populations, small communities, and rural areas.

A total of $500 million is to be transferred by the Secretary from the Federal Hospital Insurance Trust Fund and the Federal Supplementary Medical Insurance Trust Fund for this program. The Secretary has the authority to continue or expand the scope and duration of the program if it were determined that quality of care would improve and projected Medicare spending could be reduced. *The CBO score is $0.3 billion for FY2010-FY2014 and $0.5 billion for FY2010-FY2019.*

Sec. 3027. Extension of Gainsharing Demonstration. Certain gainsharing demonstrations to evaluate arrangements between hospitals and physicians have been authorized. CMS is currently operating two projects, each consisting of one hospital in New York and West Virginia. Although authorized to begin on January 1, 2007, the project began on October 1, 2008, and was scheduled to end on December 31, 2009. The Secretary was required to submit mandated reports by certain due dates. The project was appropriated $6 million in FY2006 to be available for expenditure through FY2010. Under this provision of PPACA, the authority to conduct the gainsharing demonstration project in operation as of October 1, 2008 will be extended until September 30, 2011. The due date of the required interim report is extended from December 1, 2008, to March 31, 2011, with the final report due on March 31, 2013. An additional $1.6 million is to be appropriated in FY2010; all appropriations are available through FY2014 or until expended. *The CBO score is $0.0 billion for FY2010-FY2014 and $0.0 billion for FY2010-FY2019.*

Subtitle B—Improving Medicare for Patients and Providers

Part I—Ensuring Beneficiary Access to Physician Care and Other Services

Sec. 3101. Increase in the Physician Payment Update ***removed by Sec. 10310.***[39]

Sec. 3102, as modified by Sec. 1108 of the Reconciliation Act. Extension of the Work Geographic Index Floor and Revisions to the Practice Expense Geographic Adjustment Under the Medicare Physician Fee Schedule. The Medicare fee schedule is adjusted geographically for three factors to reflect differences in the cost of resources needed to produce physician services: physician work, practice expense, and medical malpractice insurance. The geographic adjustments are indices—known as Geographic Practice Cost Indices (GPCIs)—that reflect how each area compares to the national average in a "market basket" of goods. A value of 1.00 represents an average across all areas. A series of bills set a temporary floor value of 1.00 on the physician work index beginning January 2004; most recently, Section 134 of the MIPPA extended the application of this floor when calculating Medicare physician reimbursement through December, 2009. The other geographic indices (for practice expense and medical malpractice) were not modified by these acts.

This provision provides a short extension of the floor and introduces a new methodology to determine the practice expense GPCI. First, the provision extends the 1.00 floor for the geographic index for physician work for an additional year through December 31, 2010. Second, the provision directs the Secretary to adjust the practice expense GPCI for 2010 and 2011 to reflect 1/2 of the difference between the relative costs of employee wages and rents in each of the different fee schedule areas and the national averages (i.e., a blend of 1/2 local and 1/2 national) instead of the full difference under current law. Relief applies only to areas with a practice expense GPCI less than 1.0. The provision holds harmless any areas negatively impacted by the adjustment.

The provision directs the Secretary to analyze current methods of establishing practice expense geographic adjustments under the physician fee schedule (PE GPCI) and evaluate data that fairly and reliably establishes distinctions in the costs of operating a medical practice in the different Medicare payment localities. Based on the analysis and evaluation, the Secretary is to make appropriate adjustments to the PE GPCI to ensure accurate geographic adjustments across payment areas, no later than January 1, 2012. Adjustments made in 2012 are to be made without regard to the adjustments made in 2010 and 2011. If the Secretary has not completed the required analysis and evaluation and made appropriate adjustments in the Medicare Physician Fee Schedule rule for 2012 (or subsequent year), the 2011 payment rule would remain in effect. *CBO estimates that this provision will cost a total of $2.2 billion over the next three years with no further impact over the remaining years of the 10-year budget window.*

Sec. 3103. Extension of Exceptions Process for Medicare Therapy Caps. Current law places two annual per beneficiary payment limits for all outpatient therapy services provided by non-hospital providers. For 2009, the annual limit on the allowed amount for outpatient physical therapy and speech-language pathology combined is $1,840, and there is a separate limit for occupational therapy of $1,840. The Secretary was required to implement an exceptions process for 2006, 2007, and the first half of 2008 for cases in which the provision of additional therapy services was determined to be medically necessary. Section 141 of MIPPA extended the exceptions process for therapy caps through December 31, 2009. The Temporary Extension Act of 2010, H.R. 4691 extended the exceptions process through March 31, 2010. This provision of PPACA extends the exceptions process for therapy caps through December 31, 2010. *CBO estimates that this provision will cost a total of $800 million over the next two years, with no additional impact over the remaining years of the 10-year budget window.*

Sec. 3104. Extension of Payment for Technical Component of Certain Physician Pathology Services. In 1999, the Health Care Financing Administration, (now the Centers for Medicare and Medicaid Services or CMS), proposed terminating an exception to a payment rule that had permitted laboratories to receive direct payment from Medicare when providing technical pathology services that had been outsourced by certain hospitals. This exception has been extended through legislation at various times. Most recently, the Medicare Modernization Act of 2003 (MMA, P.L. 108-173) extended the provision until January 1, 2010. This proposal extends the provision until January 1, 2011. *CBO estimates that this provision will cost $100 million in 2010, with negligible or zero costs in future years.*

Sec. 3105 as modified by Sec. 10311. Extension of Ambulance Add-ons. Bonus payments were established for ground ambulance services furnished on or after July 1, 2004, and before January 1, 2010, that originate in a qualified rural area. The qualified rural areas are those with the lowest population densities that collectively represent a total of 25% of the population. Subsequently, the Medicare rate for ground ambulance services otherwise established for the year was increased an additional 3% for rural ambulance services and 2% for other areas for the period July 1, 2008, through December 31, 2009. Areas designated as rural on December 31, 2006, are treated as rural for purposes of payments for air ambulance services during this period as well. This provision extends the bonus payments and the increased ground ambulance payments until January 1, 2011. The provision to pay certain urban air ambulance services as rural is extended until January 1, 2011, as well. *The CBO score is $0.1 billion for FY2010-FY2014 and $0.1 billion for FY2010-FY2019.*

Sec. 3106 as modified by 10312. Extension of Certain Payment Rules for Long-term Care Hospital Services and of Moratorium on the Establishment of Certain Hospitals and Facilities. Long-term care hospitals (LTCHs) are designed to provide extended medical and rehabilitative care for patients who are clinically complex and have multiple acute or chronic conditions. LTCHs that are distinct part units of other hospitals are not explicitly permitted by the Medicare statute. Over time, however, the LTCH industry has evolved to include co-located hospitals-within-hospitals (HwHs) or satellite facilities in addition to traditional freestanding facilities. CMS has implemented additional organizational requirements on these LTCHs, in an attempt to ensure that these are separate entities. Certain

LTCHs (grandfathered HwHs) have been exempted from the requirements. Starting October 1, 2004, CMS established limits on the number of discharged Medicare patients that an HwHs and satellite LTCHs (except grandfathered LTCHs) can admit and be paid as independent LTCHs; after that threshold has been reached, generally, the LTCH will receive a substantially lower payment for subsequent patient admissions who have been discharged from the host hospital. Starting July 1, 2007, CMS extended this payment policy to other types of LTCHs, including grandfathered entities. Congress provided for a three-year moratorium on the application of this payment policy for certain LTCHs starting December 29, 2007.

Effective for the first cost reporting period beginning on or after October 1, 2002, LTCHs are paid according to a prospective payment system (PPS), subject to a five-year transition period. By statute, total payments under LTCH-PPS must be equal to the amount that would have been paid if the PPS had not been implemented in the initial year of implementation. CMS proposed to review LTCH payments and make a one-time prospective adjustment to the LTCH PPS to correct for any errors in the original budget neutrality calculations. The same moratorium was applied to this policy.

The LTCH-PPS includes certain case level adjustments for short stay and interrupted stay cases. CMS adopted a very short-stay outlier payment policy starting July 1, 2007 to reduce payments for patients who have lengths of stay that are less than or equal to one standard deviation from the geometric average length-of-stay of the same MS-DRG under the IPPS. The same moratorium was applied to this policy. Finally, a three-year moratorium on new LTCHs, including HwHs and satellite facilities, and on the increase of hospital beds in existing LTCHs was established.

This PPACA provision extends the existing three-year moratoriums for two years until December 29, 2012. *The CBO score is $0.2 billion for FY2010-FY2014 and $0.2 billion for FY2010-FY2019.*

Sec. 3107. Extension of Physician Fee Schedule Mental Health Add-On. The Medicare Improvements for Patients and Providers Act of 2008 (MIPPA, P.L. 110-275) increased payments for certain Medicare mental health services by 5% beginning on July 1, 2008 and ending on December 31, 2009. This provision extends the add-on payment provision through December 31, 2010. *The CBO score is $0.0 billion for FY2010-FY2014 and $0.0 billion for FY2010-FY2019.*

Sec. 3108. Permitting Physician Assistants to Order Post-Hospital Extended Care Services. In a skilled nursing facility (SNF), Medicare law allows physicians, as well as nurse practitioners and clinical nurse specialists who do not have a direct or indirect employment relationship with a SNF, but who are working in collaboration with a physician, to certify the need for post-hospital extended care services for purposes of Medicare payment. Section 20.2.1 of Chapter 8 of the Medicare Benefit Policy Manual defines post-hospital extended care services as services provided as an extension of care for a condition for which the individual received inpatient hospital services. Extended care services are considered "post-hospital" if they are initiated within 30 days after discharge from a hospital stay that included at least three consecutive days of medically necessary inpatient hospital care.

This PPACA provision will allow a physician assistant who does not have a direct or indirect employment relationship with a SNF, but who is working in collaboration with a physician, to certify the need for post-hospital extended care services for Medicare payment purposes, beginning on or after January 1, 2011. *The CBO score is $0.0 billion for FY2010-FY2014 and $0.0 billion for FY2010-FY2019.*

Sec. 3109. Exemption of Certain Pharmacies from Accreditation Requirements. MMA required the Secretary to establish and implement quality standards for suppliers of durable medical equipment, prosthetics and supplies (DMEPOS) under Part B of Medicare. MIPPA required DMEPOS suppliers to prove their compliance with the quality standards by being accredited by October 1, 2009; P.L. 111-72 extended the deadline for pharmacies to obtain accreditation to before January 1, 2010. In general, MIPPA exempted specified eligible professionals from having to comply with the accreditation requirements. Pharmacists and pharmacies are not exempted from the accreditation requirements. PPACA extends to January 1, 2011, the accreditation deadline for all pharmacies not participating in competitive bidding. Effective January 1, 2011, PPACA exempts certain pharmacies from the accreditation requirements, although all pharmacies will still be required to meet accreditation requirements to qualify for competitive bidding. A pharmacy will be exempt from the accreditation requirements if the pharmacy (1) submits an attestation that its total Medicare DMEPOS billings represent less than 5% of total pharmacy sales for the previous three-year period, or other period as specified by the Secretary; (2) submits an attestation that it has been enrolled as a provider of DMEPOS under Medicare for at least five years with no final adverse determinations against it for the past five years; and (3) is willing to submit documentation to the Secretary (based on a random sample of pharmacies) that would allow the Secretary to verify the above information. The documentation is to consist of an accountant certification or filing of tax returns by the pharmacy. However, PPACA allows the Secretary to create a more appropriate alternative accreditation requirement and apply the alternative requirement to all pharmacies. *The CBO score is $0.0 billion for FY2010-FY2014 and $0.0 billion for FY2010-FY2019.*

Sec. 3110. Part B Special Enrollment Period for Disabled Tricare Beneficiaries. TRICARE, the health care plan under the Department of Defense (DOD) that covers members of the uniformed services, their families and survivors, was extended to Medicare-eligible military retirees, their Medicare-eligible spouses and dependent children and Medicare-eligible widow/widowers by the Floyd D. Spence National Defense Authorization Act of 2001 (P.L. 106-398). This law authorized a program known as TRICARE For Life (TFL) which acts as a secondary payer to Medicare and provides supplemental coverage to TRICARE-eligible beneficiaries who are entitled to Medicare Part A based on age, disability or end stage renal disease (ESRD). In order to participate in TFL, these TRICARE-eligible beneficiaries must enroll in and pay premiums for Medicare Part B. Under Present Law (10 U.S.C. 1086(d)), TRICARE-eligible beneficiaries who are entitled to Medicare Part A based on age, disability or ESRD, but decline Part B, lose eligibility for TRICARE benefits. Additionally, individuals who choose not to enroll in Medicare Part B upon becoming eligible may elect to do so later during an annual enrollment period; however, the Medicare Part B late enrollment penalty, would apply. Veterans' advocacy groups have reported that many beneficiaries are not aware that their TRICARE coverage is dependent upon Part B enrollment.

This provision creates a twelve-month special enrollment period (SEP) for military retirees, their spouses (including widows/ widowers) and dependent children, who are otherwise eligible for TRICARE and entitled to Medicare Part A based on disability or ESRD, but who have declined Part B. This twelve-month special enrollment period (SEP) will be available to individuals once in their lifetime and begin on the day after the last day of the initial enrollment period. Individuals will also have the option of choosing Part B coverage retroactive to the first month after the initial enrollment period. The late enrollment penalty will not apply to individuals who enroll during the SEP. The Secretary of Defense is required to identify and notify individuals of their eligibility for the SEP; the Secretary of Health and Human Services and the Commissioner for Social Security are to support these efforts. This provision is effective on the date of enactment. *The CBO score is $0.0 billion for FY2010-FY2014 and $0.0 billion for FY2010-FY2019.*

Sec. 3111. Payment for Bone Density Tests. Dual energy X-ray absorptiometry (DXA) machines are used to measure bone mass to identify individuals who may have or be at risk of having osteoporosis. For those individuals who are eligible, Medicare will pay for a bone density study once every two years, or more frequently if the procedure is determined to be medically necessary. As reported by CMS and MedPAC, spending for imaging services reimbursed under the Medicare physician fee schedule grew rapidly between 2003 and 2005. The Deficit Reduction Act of 2005 (DRA; P.L. 109-171) capped reimbursement of the technical component for x-ray and imaging services at the lesser rate of the hospital outpatient rate or the physician fee schedule. Additionally, CMS implemented a new methodology for determining resource-based practice expense payments for all services that has led to reductions in the professional component reimbursement. It is estimated that reimbursement rates for DXA services have been reduced by more than half since 2006. This provision sets payments for DXA at 70% of the 2006 reimbursement rates for these services in 2010 and 2011. The provision also directs the Secretary to arrange with the Institute of Medicine of the National Academies to study and report to the Secretary and Congress on the ramifications of Medicare reimbursement reductions for DXA on beneficiary access to bone mass measurement benefits. *CBO estimates that this provision will cost $0.1 billion in each of FY2010 and FY2011.*

Sec. 3112. Revision to the Medicare Improvement Fund. Section 188 of MIPPA established the Medicare Improvement Fund (MIF), available to the Secretary to make improvements under the original fee-for-service program under Parts A and B for Medicare beneficiaries. Under prior law, $22.3 billion was available for services furnished during FY2014. The provision will eliminate the funding in the MIF. *The CBO score is -$15.6 billion for FY2010-FY2014 and is -$20.7 billion for FY2010-FY2019.*

Sec. 3113. Treatment of Certain Complex Diagnostic Laboratory Tests. Currently, Medicare reimbursement for diagnostic laboratory tests performed on specimens collected from a hospital patient is included in the hospital payment (DRG or outpatient PPS). The provision requires the establishment of a demonstration project under Medicare Part B that will make separate payments to laboratories for complex diagnostic laboratory tests provided to Medicare beneficiaries.

The term ''complex diagnostic laboratory test'' means a diagnostic laboratory test that is (1) an analysis of gene protein expression, topographic genotyping, or a cancer chemotherapy sensitivity assay; (2) determined by the Secretary to be a laboratory test for which there is not an alternative test having equivalent performance characteristics; (3) billed using a Health Care Procedure Coding System (HCPCS) code other than a not otherwise classified code; (4) approved or cleared by the Food and Drug Administration or is covered under the Medicare program; and (5) described in section 1861(s)(3) of the Social Security Act (42 U.S.C. 1395x(s)(3)). The term "separate payment" means direct payment to a laboratory (including a hospital-based or independent laboratory) that performs a complex diagnostic laboratory test on a specimen collected from a hospital patient if the test is performed after the hospitalization and if a separate Medicare payment would not otherwise be made.

The demonstration project is to run for a two-year period beginning on July 1, 2011, so long as the cost of the demonstration program does not exceed $100 million. Not later than two years after the completion of the demonstration project, the Secretary is required to submit a report to Congress that includes (1) an assessment of the impact of the demonstration project on access to care, quality of care, health outcomes, and expenditures or savings to the Medicare program, and (2) such recommendations as the Secretary would determine to be appropriate. *CBO estimates that this provision will cost a total of $100 million over the next 5 years with no additional impact over the remaining years of the 10-year budget window.*

Sec. 3114. Improved Access for Certified Nurse-Midwife Services. Section 1833 of the SSA provides for Medicare payments for services received by covered individuals. For certified nurse-midwife services, the amount required to be paid is 80% of the lesser of either (1) the actual charge for the services, or (2) the amount determined by a fee schedule established by the Secretary. The fee schedule is not allowed to exceed 65% of the prevailing charge that would be allowed for the same services performed by a physician. This provision amends Section 1833 by adding that for services provided on or after January 1, 2011, the fee schedule for certified-midwife services will not be allowed to exceed 100% of the fee schedule amount provided under Section 1848 for the same service performed by a physician. *The CBO score is $0.0 billion for FY2010-FY2014 and $0.0 billion for FY2010-FY2019.*

Sec. 10323. Medicare Coverage for Individuals Exposed to Environmental Health Hazards. To be eligible for Medicare, one must be (1) 65 years or older and eligible to receive Social Security; or (2) under 65, permanently disabled, and have received Social Security disability insurance payments for at least two years; or (3) have Amyotrophic Lateral Sclerosis (ALS-Lou Gehrig's disease); or (4) have end-stage renal disease (ESRD). This provision will provide Medicare coverage and medical screening services to certain individuals exposed to environmental health hazards. An individual with one or more specified lung diseases or types of cancer who lived for 6 months during a specified period prior to diagnosis in an area subject to a public health emergency declaration by the Environmental Protection Agency (EPA) as of June 17, 2009, is be deemed entitled to benefits under Part A and eligible to enroll in Part B. The Secretary is required to establish a pilot program, with appropriate reimbursement methodologies, to provide comprehensive, coordinated, and cost-effective care to such individuals who enroll in Part B. Further, the Secretary has the authority to so deem any other individual diagnosed with an illness caused by an environmental hazard to which an EPA emergency declaration applies who lived for 6 months in the affected area during a period determined by the Secretary. There is to be appropriated $23 million for the period FY2010 through FY2014, and $20 million for each 5-fiscal year period thereafter, to carry out the screening and public information dissemination program. *The CBO score is $0.1 billion for FY2010-FY2014 and $0.3 billion for FY2010-FY2019.*

Sec. 10336. GAO Study and Report on Medicare Beneficiary Access to High-Quality Dialysis Services The Medicare Improvements for Patients and Providers Act of 2008 (MIPPA, P.L. 110-275) requires the Secretary to implement a bundled payment system, making a single payment for Medicare renal dialysis services, to be phased in over four years beginning January 1, 2011. The bundled payment will include (1) items and services included in the composite rate as of December 31, 2010; (2) erythropoiesis stimulating agents for the treatment of ESRD; (3) injectable biologicals and medications that were paid for separately under Part B, (before bundling) and any oral equivalent to such medications; and (4) diagnostic laboratory tests and other items and services furnished to individuals for the treatment of ESRD. This section of PPACA requires the Comptroller General to conduct a study and submit a report, within a year of enactment, on the impact on Medicare beneficiary access to high-quality dialysis services of including specified oral drugs that are furnished to beneficiaries for the treatment of ESRD and included in the ESRD bundled prospective payment system. The study is to include an analysis of (1) the ability of providers of services and renal dialysis facilities to furnish specified oral drugs; (2) the ability of providers of services and renal dialysis facilities to comply with applicable State laws, such as State pharmacy licensure requirements in order to furnish such drugs; (3) whether appropriate quality measures exist to safeguard care for Medicare beneficiaries being furnished specified oral drugs by providers of services and renal dialysis facilities; and (4) other areas determined appropriate by the Comptroller General. *The CBO score is $0.0 billion for FY2010-FY2014 and $0.0 billion for FY2010-FY2019.*

Part II—Rural Protections

Sec. 3121. Extension of Outpatient Hold Harmless Provision. Small rural hospitals (with no more than 100 beds) that are not sole community hospitals (SCHs) can receive additional Medicare payments if their outpatient payments under the prospective payment system are less than under the prior hospital outpatient department (HOPD) reimbursement system. For calendar year (CY) 2006, these hospitals received 95% of the difference between payments under the prospective payment system and those that would have been made under the prior reimbursement system. The hospitals received 90% of the difference in CY2007 and 85% of the difference in CY2008 and CY2009. Sole community hospitals with not more than 100 beds received 85% of the payment difference for covered HOPD services furnished on or after January 1, 2009, and before January 1, 2010. The provision establishes that small rural hospitals are to receive 85% of the payment difference in CY2010. SCHs with not more than 100 beds will receive 85% of the payment difference in CY2010. The 100-bed limitation for SCHs is removed so that all SCHs are receiving 85% of the payment difference in CY2010. *The CBO score is $0.2 billion for FY2010-FY2014 and $0.2 billion for FY2010-FY2019.*

Sec. 3122. Extension of Medicare Reasonable Costs Payments for Certain Clinical Diagnostic Laboratory Tests Furnished to Hospital Patients in Certain Rural Areas.[40] Generally, hospitals that provide clinical diagnostic laboratory services under Part B are reimbursed using a fee schedule. Hospitals with under 50 beds in qualified rural areas (certain rural areas with low population densities) receive 100% of reasonable cost reimbursement for the clinical diagnostic laboratories covered under Part B that are provided as outpatient hospital services. Reasonable cost reimbursement for laboratory services provided by these hospitals ended July 1, 2008. Under this provision, reasonable cost reimbursement for clinical diagnostic laboratory service for qualifying rural hospitals with under 50 beds will be reinstated from July 1, 2010 and extended for one year, ending July 1, 2011. *The CBO score is $0.0 billion for FY2010-FY2014 and $0.0 billion for FY2010-FY2019.*

Sec. 3123 as modified by Sec. 10313. Extension of the Rural Community Hospital Demonstration Program. CMS is conducting a five-year Rural Community Hospital Demonstration Program to test the feasibility and advisability of reasonable cost reimbursement for small rural hospitals (those with fewer than 51 beds) in low population density areas. No more than 15 hospitals can participate in the demonstration. Currently, there are 10 hospitals participating in the program. This provision extends the demonstration program for an additional five years, expands the maximum number of participating hospitals to 30 for that period, and specifies that the 20 states with low population densities will participate in the demonstration project. The Secretary is to provide for the continued participation for those hospitals that are in the demonstration at the end of the initial five-year period during the five-year extension unless the hospital elects to discontinue such participation. Participants will receive the reasonable cost for discharges occurring in the first cost reporting period beginning on or after the first day of the five-year extension. *The CBO score is $0.0 billion for FY2010-FY2014 and $0.0 billion for FY2010-FY2019.*

Sec. 3124. Extension of the Medicare-Dependent Hospital (MDH) Program. Medicare dependent hospitals (MDHs) are small rural hospitals with a high proportion of patients who are Medicare beneficiaries. Specifically, the hospitals have at least 60% of acute inpatient days or discharges attributable to Medicare in FY1987 or in 2 of the 3 most recently audited cost reporting periods. As specified in regulation, they cannot be a sole community hospital and must have 100 or fewer beds. MDHs receive special treatment, including higher payments, under Medicare's inpatient prospective payment system. The sunset date for the MDH classification has been periodically extended by legislation and was set to expire September 30, 2011. Under this provision, the MDH classification is extended one year, until September 30, 2012. *The CBO score is $0.0 billion for FY2010-FY2014 and $0.0 billion for FY2010-FY2019.*

Sec. 3125 as modified by 10314. Temporary Improvements to the Medicare Inpatient Hospital Payment Adjustment for Low-Volume Hospitals. Under Medicare's inpatient prospective payment system (IPPS), certain low-volume hospitals receive a payment adjustment to account for their higher costs per discharge. A low-volume hospital is defined as an acute care hospital that is located more than 25 road miles from another comparable hospital and that has less than 800 total discharges during the fiscal year. The Secretary is required to determine an appropriate percentage increase for these low-volume hospitals based on the empirical relationship between the standardized cost-per-case for such hospitals and their total discharges to account for the additional incremental costs (if any) that are associated with such number of discharges. The low-volume adjustment is limited to no more than 25%. Accordingly, under regulations, qualifying hospitals (those located more than 25 road miles from another comparable hospital) with less than 200 total discharges receive a 25% payment increase for every Medicare discharge.

Under this provision, a temporary adjustment that would increase payment in FY2011 and FY2012 for certain low-volume hospitals will be created. A low volume hospital could be located more than 15 road miles from another comparable hospital and have 1,600 discharges of individuals entitled to or enrolled for Medicare Part A benefits. The Secretary is to determine the applicable percentage increase using a continuous linear sliding scale ranging from 25% for low-volume hospitals with 200 or fewer discharges of individuals with Medicare Part A benefits to no adjustment for hospitals with greater than 1,600 discharges of individuals with Medicare Part A benefits. *The CBO score is $0.0 billion for FY2010-FY2014 and $0.3 billion for FY2010-FY2019.*

Sec. 3126. Improvements to the Demonstration Project on Community Health Integration Models in Certain Rural Counties. A demonstration project to allow eligible entities to develop and test new models for the delivery of health care services in eligible counties has been authorized. Those eligible to participate in the demonstration project are limited to certain entities in States with at least 65% of its counties in the State with 6 or fewer residents per square mile. Based on these criteria, the Secretary is instructed to select up to 4 states to participate in the demonstration program, and within those states, up to 6 counties. For a county to be eligible to participate, it must have 6 or fewer residents per square mile and contain a critical access hospital (CAH) that furnished one or more of specified services (home health, hospice, or rural health clinic) and had a daily inpatient census of 5 or less as of date of enactment; skilled nursing facility services must be available in the eligible county. The three-year demonstration project is to begin on October 1, 2009, and be done in a budget neutral manner. This section of PPACA eliminates the limit of 6 eligible counties that may participate in the demonstration project within the qualifying states. Rural health clinic services will no longer be one of specified CAH services. Rural health clinic services are removed from the definition of other essential services and replaced with physician services. *The CBO score is $0.0 billion for FY2010-FY2014 and $0.0 billion for FY2010-FY2019.*

Sec. 3127. MedPAC Study on Adequacy of Medicare Payments for Health Care Providers Serving in Rural Areas. Under this provision, MedPAC is required to review payment adequacy for rural health care providers and suppliers serving the Medicare program and provide a report to Congress by January 1, 2011. MedPAC is to analyze rural payment adjustments, beneficiaries' access to care in rural communities, adequacy of Medicare payments to rural providers and suppliers, and quality of care in rural areas, and submit a report to Congress by January 1, 2011. *The CBO score is $0.0 billion for FY2010-FY2014 and $0.0 billion for FY2010-FY2019.*

Sec. 3128. Technical Correction Related to Critical Access Hospital Services. Critical Access Hospitals (CAHs) are limited-service rural facilities that meet certain distance criteria;

offer 24-hour emergency care; have no more than 25 acute care inpatient beds and have a 96-hour average length of stay. Generally, a rural hospital designated as a CAH receives 101% reasonable, cost based reimbursement for inpatient and outpatient care rendered to Medicare beneficiaries. A CAH may elect an all-inclusive outpatient payment which is equal to a 101% of reasonable costs for facility services plus 115% of the Medicare physician fee schedule payment for professional services when the physician or practitioner has reassigned his or her billing rights to the CAH. As part of its FY2010 rulemaking process, starting October 1, 2009, CMS will lower the facility component of the all-inclusive, elective payment method from 101% to 100% of the CAH's reasonable costs; the payment for professional services will remain at 115% of the fee schedule amount. Medicare pays for ambulance services provided by a CAH or by an entity owned and operated by a CAH at 100% of reasonable costs, but only if CAH or the entity is the only supplier or provider of ambulance services with a 35-mile drive of the CAH or the entity.

Under this provision, Medicare will pay the facility component of the all-inclusive elective CAH payment for outpatient services at 101% of reasonable costs. Medicare will pay for qualifying ambulance services provided by a CAH or by an entity owned and operated by a CAH at 101% of reasonable cost. *The CBO score is $0.0 billion for FY2010-FY2014 and $0.0 billion for FY2010-FY2019.*

Sec. 3129. Extension of and Revisions to Medicare Rural Hospital Flexibility Program. One component of the Medicare Rural Hospital Flexibility Program is a grant program (FLEX grants) that is administered by the Health Resources and Services Administration (HRSA). Under this program, Flex grants may be awarded to States and to small rural hospital for certain purposes. There are certain limitations imposed on the use of grant funds for administrative expenses, both at the state and Federal level. The FLEX grant program is authorized at $55 million for each fiscal year from 2009 and 2010 and the new rural mental health and other services grants would be authorized at $55 million for each of fiscal years 2009 and 2010. Under this provision, the FLEX grant program will be extended two years until 2012. Starting January 1, 2010, grant funding will be available to be used to assist small rural hospitals to participate in delivery system reforms made by this legislation. *The CBO score is $0.0 billion for FY2010-FY2014 and $0.0 billion for FY2010-FY2019.*[41]

Sec. 10324. Protections for Frontier States. Under this provision, starting for discharges on October 1, 2010, the area wage index of a hospital located in a frontier state (where 50% of the counties have less than six people per square mile) will be no less than one. This will not apply to states where hospitals receive an adjustment to their non-labor related share. This provision will not be applied on a budget neutral basis. The same provisions will apply to covered HOPD services furnished after January 1, 2011, in frontier states. A floor of one on the practice expense index will be established for physician services in these frontier states for physician services on or after January 1, 2011. *The CBO score is $0.8 billion for FY2010-FY2014 and $2.0 billion for FY2010-FY2019.*

Part III—Improving Payment Accuracy

Sec. 3131 as modified by Sec. 10315. Payment Adjustments for Home Health Care. Home health agencies (HHAs) are paid under a prospective payment system (PPS) that provides payments based on 60-day episodes of care for beneficiaries, subject to several adjustments. The base payment amount of the PPS is adjusted for differences in the care needs of patients (case mix) using "HH resource groups" (HHRGs) and outlier adjustments (to account for extraordinarily costly patients), among other adjustments. Presently, there is no difference between urban and rural base payment amounts.

In CY2008, refinements to the Medicare HH PPS included, among other changes, a reduction in the payment rate for four years (to continue through CY2011) to adjust for increases in case mix that are related to changes in coding instead of increased patient severity of illness. The final CMS rule for CY2010 continues with the 2.75% reduction to the HH PPS rates for CY2010. This reduction is consistent with the CMS proposed and final rules for CY2008 explaining that changes to calculations of case mix would result in a four-year adjustment to payment rates, including an adjustment downward for 60-day episode of care of 2.75% for CYs 2008, 2009, and 2010, and 2.71% for CY2011. Among other things, the final rule also implements a cap on outlier payments (i.e., payments for unusually costly 60-day episodes of care) at 10% of total payments per HHA, and no more than 2.5% of total aggregate PPS payments for all of HH.

Under PPACA, starting in CY2014, the Secretary will be required to rebase home health payments by a percentage considered appropriate by the Secretary to, among other things, reflect the number, mix and level of intensity of HH services in an episode, and the average cost of providing care. In doing so, the Secretary may consider the differences between HH agencies in regards to hospital-based and freestanding providers; for-profit and non-profit providers; and resource costs between urban and rural providers. Any adjustments that result must be made before the annual payment updates are applied for that year. A four-year phase-in, ending in 2017, will be implemented, in equal increments; each increment may not exceed 3.5% of the HH PPS base payment amount as of the date of enactment.

Regarding payments, the Secretary is required to reduce the standard HHRG amounts such that the aggregate reduction in payments will equal 5% of total PPS payments for a period. And, similar to the CMS final rule for CY2010, the total amount of additional payments for outliers may not exceed 2.5% of the total PPS payments in a given fiscal year (or calendar year). Also similar to the CMS final rule, starting in CY2011 the Secretary is required to establish a provider-specific annual cap of 10% of revenues that a HH agency may be reimbursed in a given year from outlier payments. For visits ending on or after April 1, 2010, and before January 1, 2016, the Secretary is directed to provide for a 3% add-on payment for HH providers serving rural areas.

The provision also requires MedPAC to conduct a study on the implementation of the HH payment adjustment under the rebasing, including an analysis of its impact on access to care, quality outcomes, the number of HH agencies, rural agencies, urban agencies, for-profit agencies, and nonprofit agencies. MedPAC must submit to Congress a report on this study, together with recommendations for legislation and administrative action no later than January 1, 2015.

No later than March 1, 2014, the Secretary is required to submit a study (after consulting with appropriate stakeholders) to Congress on HH agency costs involved with providing ongoing access to care to low-income Medicare beneficiaries or beneficiaries in medically underserved areas, and in treating beneficiaries with varying levels of severity of illness. In conducting the study, the Secretary could analyze methods to potentially revise the home health PPS to account for costs related to patient severity of illness or improvements in beneficiary access to care. Examples may include (1) payment adjustments for services involving additional or fewer resources; (2) changes reflecting resources involved in providing HH services to low-income Medicare beneficiaries or those residing in medically underserved areas; (3) ways outlier payments may be revised to reflect costs of treating Medicare beneficiaries with high levels of severity of illness; and (4) other issues determined appropriate by the Secretary. In conducting the study, the Secretary could also analyze operational issues involved with potential implementation of revisions to the home health payment system, including impacts on both home health agencies and administrative and systems issues for CMS. It could also, among other factors, evaluate whether additional research is needed.

Taking into account this study's results, the Secretary may provide for a four-year demonstration, beginning no later than January 1, 2015, to test whether payment adjustments for HH services would substantially improve access to care for patients with high severity of illness, or low income or underserved Medicare beneficiaries. The Secretary may not reduce standard PPS amounts to offset any increase in payments from the demonstration during that or subsequent periods. The Secretary will also be required to conduct an evaluation of the project, and submit a report to Congress, by a date specified by the Secretary.

The Secretary is to provide for the transfer from the Federal Hospital Insurance Trust Fund and the Federal Supplementary Medical Insurance Trust Fund, in the proportion as the Secretary determines appropriate, of $500 million for the period of fiscal years 2015 through 2018. Such funds are to be made available for the study, as well as for the design, implementation, and evaluation of the demonstration. Amounts are available until expended. *The CBO score is -$4.2 billion for FY2010-FY2014 and -$39.7 billion for FY2010-FY2019 and includes the effect of Sec. 3401 related to a productivity adjustment.*

Sec. 3132. Hospice Reform. For a person to be considered terminally ill for eligibility purposes for Medicare's hospice benefit, the beneficiary's attending physician and the medical director of the hospice (or physician member of the hospice team) must certify that the individual has a life expectancy of six months or less. The medical director or physician member of the hospice team must recertify that the beneficiary is terminally ill at the beginning of each 90- or 60-day eligibility period. Medicare payments to hospices are predetermined fixed daily amounts for each case, and are based on one of four prospectively determined units of payment, which correspond to four different levels of care (i.e., routine home care, continuous home care, inpatient respite care, and general inpatient care).

Under the provision, Secretary is required to begin, by January 1, 2011, collecting additional data and information needed to revise payments for hospice care. Not earlier than October 1, 2013, the Secretary will be required to, by rulemaking, implement budget neutral revisions to the methodology for determining hospice payments for routine home care and other services that could include per diem payments to hospices reflecting differences in resources used or additional payments (end-of-episode payment) reflecting resource intensity of services provided at the end of episode, among others.

In addition, the provision requires the Secretary to impose new requirements on hospice providers that participate in Medicare, including requiring, on or after January 1, 2011, that (1) a hospice physician or advanced practice nurse have a face-to-face encounter with the individual regarding eligibility and recertification and attest that hospice visits are made; and (2) stays in excess of 180 days, that meet certain conditions, be medically reviewed by CMS or its contractors. *The CBO score is $0.0 for FY2010-FY2014 and -0.1 billion for FY2010-FY2019.*

Sec. 3133 as modified by Sec. 10316 of PPACA, and by Sec. 1041 of the Reconciliation Act. Improvement to Medicare Disproportionate Share Hospital (DSH) Payments. Medicare's disproportionate share hospital (DSH) adjustment was included in the inpatient prospective payment system (IPPS) in 1986 on the premise that low-income patients are more costly to treat and those acute care hospitals serving a large number of such patients would be likely to have higher costs for their Medicare patients than would otherwise similar institutions. Over time, as the formulas for Medicare's DSH adjustment have been changed, the justification for the higher payments has evolved and the adjustment is viewed as a way to insure access to hospital care. Medicare's DSH payments are distributed through a hospital-specific percentage increase to its prospective payment rate. In most instances, the size of a hospital's DSH adjustment would depend upon the number of patient days provided to poor Medicare patients or Medicaid patients. In its March 2007 *Report to Congress*, MedPAC found that about three-quarters of the Medicare DSH payments (accounting for about $5.5 billion in FY2004) was not empirically justified in terms of higher patient care costs. Also, Medicare's DSH payments were poorly targeted to hospitals' shares of uncompensated care

Under this provision, starting in FY2014 and for subsequent fiscal years, the Secretary will make DSH payments equal to 25% of what otherwise would be made, a payment that represents the empirically justified amount as determined by MedPAC in its March 2007 *Report to Congress.* In addition to this amount, starting in FY2014, the Secretary will pay to such acute care hospitals an additional amount using a formula that is the product of three factors:

- The difference in the hospital's DSH payments because of this legislation.
- For FY2014, the difference in the percentage change in the uninsured under-65 population from 2013 (as calculated from current estimates from CBO data before the vote to enroll the Act in the House) and those who are uninsured in the most recent period for which data is available minus 0.1 percentage points; in FY2015 through FY2019, there will be a 0.2 percentage point subtraction; in FY2018 and subsequently, the calculation will use data from the Census Bureau or other appropriate sources as certified by the Chief Actuary of CMS.
- The percentage of uncompensated care provided by the hospital (relative to all acute care hospitals) for a selected period based on appropriate data.

There will be no administrative or judicial review of any estimate used to determine the factors or any periods used to establish the factors. *The CBO score is $0.0 billion for FY2010-FY2014 and -$22.1 billion for FY2010-FY2019.*

Sec. 3134. Misvalued Codes Under the Physician Fee Schedule. The Medicare physician fee schedule is based on assigning relative weights to each of the more than 7,000 physician service codes used to bill Medicare. The relative value for a service compares the relative work involved in performing one service with the work involved in providing other physicians' services. The scale used to compare the value of one service with another is known as a resource-based relative value scale (RBRVS). CMS is responsible for maintaining and updating the fee schedule, including the modification and refinement of the methodology for estimating relative value units (RVUs). CMS relies on advice and recommendations from the American Medical Association/Specialty Society Relative Value Scale Update Committee (RUC) in its assessments. In general, as currently implemented, increases in RVUs for a service or number of services lowers the resultant fees for other physician services because of the budget neutrality condition. One consequence has been that the payments for evaluation and management codes, whose RVUs typically are not increased over time, have fallen relative to other codes whose RVUs have increased and as a consequence of new technologies that have been introduced into coverage with relatively high RVUs. CMS is required to review the RVUs no less than every five years.

Under this provision, the Secretary is required to periodically identify physician services as being potentially misvalued, and make appropriate adjustments to the relative values of such services under the Medicare physician fee schedule. To identify potentially misvalued services, the Secretary is to examine codes (and families of codes as appropriate) with the fastest growth, that have experienced substantial changes in practice expenses, for new technologies or services, that are frequently billed in conjunction with furnishing a single service, with low relative values, particularly those that are often billed multiple times for a single treatment, that have not been subject to review since the implementation of the RBRVS (the so-called 'Harvard-valued codes'), and other codes the Secretary determined to be appropriate. The Secretary is to review and make appropriate adjustments to the work relative value units under the fee schedule.

The provision also repeals Section 4505(d) of the Balanced Budget Act of 1997, which established requirements for developing new resource-based practice expense relative value units, as well as Section 1868(a) of the Social Security Act (42 U.S.C. 1395ee(a)), which established the Practicing Physicians Advisory Council, a group of physicians who meet quarterly to discuss proposed changes in regulations and carrier manual instructions related to physician services. *CBO estimates that this provision will have no impact on spending over the 5-year or 10-year budget window.*

Sec. 3135 as modified by Sec. 1107 of the Reconciliation Act. Modification of Equipment Utilization Factor for Advanced Imaging Services. Under the Medicare fee schedule, some services have separate payments for the technical component and the professional component. For example, imaging procedures generally have two parts: the actual taking of the image (the technical component), and the interpretation of the image (the professional component). Medicare pays for each of these components separately when the technical component is furnished by one provider and the professional component by another. When both components are furnished by one provider, Medicare makes a single global payment that is equal to the sum of the payment for each of the components.

CMS's method for calculating the Medicare fee schedule reimbursement rate for advanced imaging services assumed that imaging machines are operated 25 hours per week, or 50% of the time that practices are open for business. Setting the equipment use factor at a lower rate has led to higher payment for these services. Citing evidence showing that the utilization rate is 90%, rather than the 50% previously assumed, MedPAC has urged CMS to use the higher utilization rate in the calculation of fee schedule payments for advanced imaging services and CMS adopted a 90% use rate assumption in its 2010 final rule for Medicare physician payment. The PPACA and Reconciliation Act provisions change the utilization rate assumption for calculating the payment for advanced imaging equipment from 50%, as assumed in prior years, to 75% for 2011 and in subsequent years. This overrides the CMS 2010 final rule that applied a 90% use rate assumption.

According to MedPAC and the Government Accountability Office (GAO), there are opportunities to improve the efficiency of the Medicare fee schedule. In 2005, MedPAC recommended reducing certain fees to account for efficiencies and savings from the technical preparation and supplies achieved when multiple imaging services are furnished sequentially on contiguous body parts during the same visit. Starting January 1, 2006, physicians receive the full technical component fee for the highest paid imaging service in a visit, but technical component fees for additional imaging services are reduced by 25%. The provision increases the technical component payment reduction for sequential imaging services on contiguous body parts during the same visit from 25% to 50%. By January 1, 2013, the CMS Chief Actuary is to conduct and make publicly available an analysis of whether the cumulative expenditure reductions attributable to these adjustments are projected to exceed $3 billion for the period 2010 through 2019. *The CBO score is -$0.9 billion for FY2010-FY2014 and -$2.3 billion for FY2010-FY2019.*

Sec. 3136. Revision of Payment for Power-Driven Wheelchairs. Prior to enactment of PPACA, Medicare pays for new or replacement power-driven wheelchairs either through monthly rental payments during the beneficiary's period of medical need (not to exceed 13 continuous months), or, on a lump-sum basis. Rental payments for wheelchairs are statutorily determined as 10% of the purchase price of the chair for each of the first 3 months and 7.5% of the purchase price for each of the remaining 10 months of the rental period. Medicare pays for most DME on the basis of a fee schedule, except in Competitive Acquisition Areas where payments are to be determined based on supplier bids. Starting January 1, 2011, PPACA restricts the lump-sum payment option for new or replacement chairs to only the complex, rehabilitative power wheelchairs. The lump-sum payment option is eliminated for all other wheelchairs. The provision does not apply to competitive acquisition areas prior to January 1, 2011. Also starting January 1, 2011, the rental payment for power-driven wheelchairs will be 15% of the purchase price for each of the first three months (instead of 10%), and 6% of the purchase price for each of the remaining 10 months of the rental period (instead of 7.5%). *The CBO score is -$0.6 billion for FY2010-FY2014 and -$0.8 billion for FY2010-FY2019.*

Sec. 3137 as modified by Sec. 10317. Hospital Wage Index Improvement. A hospital wage index is used to adjust the standardized amount to account for the local wage variation or cost of labor in the hospital's area. Starting in FY2005, CMS has adjusted this data to account for the relative skill mix of the hospitals in the area. This occupationally mix adjusted average hourly wage is then divided by the same measure calculated using data from all hospitals in the nation to establish the area's adjusted wage index. MedPAC issued its mandated report on recommended changes to the hospital wage index in June 2007. CMS has hired an independent consulting firm to further evaluate the impact of making the recommended changes.

Unlike other providers, acute care hospitals may apply to the Medicare Geographic Classification Review Board (MGCRB) for a change in classification from a rural area to an urban area, or reassignment from one urban area to another urban area. To reclassify, a hospital had to meet certain standards, establishing that its average hourly wage (AHW) was within a certain threshold of the AHW of the area where it wanted to reclassify. Starting in FY2010, CMS raised the reclassification threshold. MGCRB hospital reclassifications are established on a budget neutral basis so aggregate inpatient payments will not increase as a result of the reclassified hospitals' higher payments.

Section 508 of the Medicare Prescription Drug, Improvement and Modernization Act of 2003 (MMA, P.L. 108-173) provided $900 million for a one-time, three year geographic reclassification of certain hospitals who were otherwise unable to qualify for administrative reclassification to areas with higher wage index values. These reclassifications were extended legislatively at various points until September 30, 2009.

This provision will extend the Section 508 reclassifications until September 30, 2010.[42] The Secretary is required to use the FY2010 wage index data (promulgated in the August 27, 2009, *Federal Register* and subsequent corrections). Beginning on April 1, 2010, the average hourly wage data of these hospitals will be included in the reclassified area only if including the data results in a higher wage index. Certain hospitals that had a lower wage index from October 1, 2009, through March 31, 2010, than from April 1, 2010, through September 30, 2010, will be paid an additional amount to reflect such difference by December 31, 2010.

By December 31, 2011, the Secretary is required to provide a plan to Congress on how to comprehensively reform the Medicare wage index system; this plan is to take into account MedPAC recommendations included in its *June 2007 Report to Congress*. The Secretary is also required to restore the reclassifications thresholds used in determining hospital reclassifications to the percentages used for FY2009 Medicare Geographic Classification Review Board (MGCRB) decisions, starting in FY2011 and in subsequent fiscal years (until the first fiscal year beginning on or after the date that is one year after the date of the submission of the Secretary's wage index reform plan). This provision is to be implemented in a budget neutral fashion. *The CBO score is $0.3 billion for FY2010-FY2014 and $0.3 billion for FY2010-FY2019.*

Sec. 3138. Treatment of Certain Cancer Hospitals. Eleven cancer hospitals are exempt from the inpatient prospective payment system (IPPS) used to pay inpatient hospital services provided by acute care hospitals. These hospitals are also held harmless under the outpatient prospective payment system (OPPS) and will not receive less from Medicare under this payment system than under the prior outpatient payment system. Under OPPS, Medicare pays for outpatient services using ambulatory payment classification (APC) groups. This provision requires the Secretary to conduct a study which would consider the cost of drugs and biologics to determine if the outpatient costs incurred by IPPS-exempt cancer hospitals with respect to Medicare's APCs exceed those costs incurred by other hospitals reimbursed under OPPS. If so, the Secretary would be required to provide for an appropriate OPPS adjustment starting January 1, 2011. *The CBO score is $0.0 billion for FY2010-FY2014 and $0.0 billion for FY2010-FY2019.*

Sec. 3139. Payment for Biosimilar Biological Products. A biologic is a preparation, such as a therapeutic product or a vaccine, which is made from living organisms. Medicare Part B pays for a limited number of drugs and therapeutic products, including biologics, administered to patients in physician offices and hospital outpatient departments, or those administered through durable medical equipment (DME) and billed by pharmacy suppliers. CMS assigns a Healthcare Common Procedure Coding System (HCPCS) code to each drug, and Medicare payments for Part B drugs are based on the average sales price (ASP) for each HCPCS code. CMS uses the same HCPCS code for all drug products listed as therapeutically equivalent in FDA's *Orange Book*. Therefore, a brand-name drug and any generic versions of the same drug would have the same HCPCS code and the prices would be averaged together for ASP determinations. The provision allows a Part B biosimilar product approved by the Food and Drug Administration to be reimbursed at the ASP of the biosimilar plus 6% of the ASP of the reference product. (The term reference biological product means the licensed biological product that is referred to in the application for the biosimilar product.) *The CBO score (Sections 3139 and Sections 7001-7003 combined) is -\$0.1 billion for FY2010-FY2014 and -\$7.1 billion for FY2010-FY2019.*[43]

Sec. 3140. Medicare Hospice Concurrent Care Demonstration Program. Medicare covers hospice care for terminally ill beneficiaries instead of most other Medicare services related to the curative treatment of their illness. The provision requires the Secretary to conduct a three-year demonstration program, from Medicare funds that would otherwise be paid for hospice care, to allow patients who are eligible for hospice to also receive all other Medicare covered services during the same period of time. The Secretary is to select not more than 15 hospice programs in both urban and rural areas to examine improvement in patient care, quality of life, and cost-effectiveness that results from the demonstration project. *The CBO score is \$0.0 billion for FY2010-FY2014 and \$0.0 billion for FY2010-FY2019.*

Sec. 3141. Application of Budget Neutrality on a National Basis in the Calculation of the Medicare Hospital Wage Index Floor for Each All-Urban and Rural State. A hospital wage index is used to adjust the standardized amount to account for the local wage variation or cost of labor in the hospital's area. As required by statute, the wage index for any urban area in a state cannot be less than the rural wage index of that state (often referred to as the rural floor). The effect of the rural floor (that is, raising the wage index for urban areas in a state to that state's rural wage index) is required to be implemented on a budget neutral basis by adjusting the wage index of all hospitals not affected by the rural floor. Until FY2009, CMS funded the budget neutrality requirement associated with the impact of the rural floor though a nationwide adjustment. Starting in FY2009, CMS began a transition to fund the budget neutrality requirement through a state-specific adjustment; the statewide adjustment would be fully implemented in FY2011. States with no hospitals receiving the rural floor wage index would not have a reduced payment; those hospitals within each state with urban areas paid at the higher rural wage index would fund the higher payments for the affected hospitals. The provision requires the application of budget neutrality requirement associated with the effect of the imputed rural and rural floor on a national basis (through a uniform, national adjustment to the area wage index) for discharges starting October 1, 2010. *The CBO score is \$0.0 billion for FY2010-FY2014 and \$0.0 billion for FY2010-FY2019.*

Sec. 3142. HHS Study on Urban Medicare-Dependent Hospitals. Medicare dependent hospitals (MDHs) are small rural hospitals with a high proportion of patients who are Medicare beneficiaries. MDHs receive special treatment, including higher payments, under Medicare's inpatient prospective payment system (IPPS). Certain other hospitals, such as rural referral centers (RRC) and sole community hospitals (SCHs) receive special treatment under IPPS. Other small, limited service critical access hospitals (CAHs) are exempt from IPPS and paid 101% of their reasonable costs. IPPS includes certain payment adjustments, such as the indirect medical education (IME) adjustment for teaching hospitals, to compensate hospitals for higher average costs which might not be in their control. The disproportionate share hospital (DSH) adjustment increases payments for hospitals that serve a relatively high proportion of poor Medicare and Medicaid patients. This provision requires the Secretary to conduct a study within 9 months of enactment on the need for an additional Medicare payments for urban Medicare-dependent hospitals paid under IPPS which receive no additional IPPS payments (have an IME or DSH adjustment) or receive special treatment (as an RRC, SCH, or MDH). CAHs are to be excluded as well. *The CBO score is $0.0 billion for FY2010-FY2014 and $0.0 billion for FY2010-FY2019.*

Sec. 3143. Protecting Home Health Benefits. This provision requires that nothing in PPACA may result in a reduction of guaranteed home health benefits under title XVIII of the Social Security Act. *CBO did not score this provision.*

Sec. 10325. Revision to Skilled Nursing Facility Prospective Payment System.[44] SNFs are paid through a PPS which is composed of a daily ("per-diem") urban or rural base payment amount that is then adjusted for case mix and area wages. The base payment is adjusted for treatment type and care needs of the beneficiary based on 53 payment-adjusted resource utilization groups (RUGs). In January 2006, CMS implemented a refined SNF PPS (using FY2001 claims data), including a parity adjustment to ensure that estimated total payments under the 53-group RUG model would maintain parity to the formerly used 44-group RUG model in a budget neutral manner.

According to the CMS final rule for FY2010, published on August 11, 2009,[45] the market basket update for FY2010 is 2.2 percentage points. In addition, CMS described how it would establish a revised case-mix classification methodology (Resource Utilization Group–Version Four; RUG-IV) and implementation schedule for FY2011 (starting October 1, 2010), reflecting updated staff time measurement data derived from the recently completed Staff Time and Resource Intensity Verification (STRIVE) project, among other things. According to CMS, these revisions to the case-mix are intended to correct for changes made for FY2006, in which changes that were intended to better account for the resources used in the care of medically complex patients resulted in payments exceeding budget neutrality estimates.

Among the changes described in the CMS FY2010 final rule are changes to the billing method for concurrent therapy. According to CMS, concurrent therapy is defined as the practice of one professional therapist treating multiple patients at the same time, each of whom can be receiving different therapy treatments. (There were previously no MDS coding restrictions regarding the number of patients that may be treated concurrently, among other things.) Prior to FY2010, SNFs were allowed to bill for concurrent therapy as individual therapy time for each patient. The FY2010 final rule requires SNFs to instead calculate the therapy minutes allocated to each individual and to report only those minutes on the MDS 3.0 for billing purposes.

The FY2010 final rule also describes changes to billing for the following high-cost staff-intensive services: ventilator/respirator, tracheostomy, suctioning, IV medications, and transfusions. Prior to the implementation of the new law, the RUG billing system accounted for the costs of these services when furnished within the prior 14 days, regardless of whether they were furnished prior to a patient's admission. According to CMS, the inclusion of these expenditures in the RUG billing system was intended to serve as a proxy for the higher-cost medically complex services delivered to certain categories of SNF residents. More recent analysis by CMS showed this to be a poor proxy for medical complexity. As a result, the FY2010 rule modifies this look-back period to include only services delivered after admission to a SNF.

PPACA makes four significant changes to the SNF PPS. First, starting in FY2012, all SNF market-basket annual updates will be subject to a productivity adjustment. Second, the Secretary is prohibited from implementing the revised case-mix classification methodology (Resource Utilization Group–Version Four; RUG-IV) described in the FY2010 final rule prior to October 1, 2011. (New CMS guidance explaining the delay of the RUG-IV implementation, as a result of PPACA, has not yet been published.) Third, the new law required the Secretary to implement the change specified in the FY2010 final rule to therapy that is furnished on a concurrent basis. Fourth, PPACA required the Secretary to implement the changes to the look-back period described in the FY2010 final rule to ensure that only those services furnished after admission to a SNF are used as factors in determining a SNF case mix classification. *The CBO score is $0.0 billion for FY2010-FY2014 and $0.0 billion for FY2010-FY2019.*

Sec. 1109 of the Reconciliation Act. Payment for Qualifying Hospitals. Medicare payments to acute care hospitals in low-cost counties will be increased by a total of $400 million for two years (FY2011 and FY2012). The qualifying hospitals are located in counties ranked in the lowest quartile of adjusted Medicare Part A and B benefit spending (adjusted by age, sex, and race). The additional payments to each qualifying hospital will be in proportion to its Medicare inpatient hospital payments relative to Medicare inpatient hospital payments for all qualifying hospitals. *The CBO score is $400 million from FY2011 through FY2012.*

Subtitle C—Provisions Relating to Part C

Sec. 3201 as modified by Sec. 10318 of PPACA and Sec. 1102 of the Reconciliation Act. Medicare Advantage Payment. Medicare Advantage (MA) is an alternative way for Medicare beneficiaries to receive covered benefits. Under MA, private plans are paid a per-person amount to provide all Medicare-covered benefits (except hospice) to beneficiaries who enroll in their plan. Payments to MA plans are determined by comparing plan bids to a benchmark. Each bid represents the plan's estimated revenue requirement for providing required Medicare services to an average Medicare beneficiary. The benchmark is the maximum amount Medicare will pay a plan. If the plan bid is below the benchmark, the plan is paid its bid plus a rebate equal to 75% of the difference between the bid and the benchmark. If the bid is above the benchmark, the plan is paid the benchmark and each plan enrollee must pay a premium equal to the difference between the bid and the benchmark. MA benchmarks are based, in part, on historical Medicare private plan payment rates. (MA benchmarks for Regional MA plans are based in part on historical MA plan payments, and in part on Regional MA plan bids.) Benchmark amounts are increased each year by the growth in Medicare spending (the national MA per capita growth percentage), or in certain years, the benchmark may be set at the greater of the previous year's rate increased by the growth in Medicare or average spending in original Medicare in that area, with adjustments. Local MA plans choose the counties they wish to serve. Regional plans must serve an entire region defined by the Secretary, and may choose to serve more than one region. Regions are made up of states or groups of states. Though all MA organizations were required to have a quality improvement program by January 1, 2010, payments to MA plans are not contingent on the quality of care provided to plan enrollees.

Under PPACA:

MA Benchmarks. Under PPACA, the benchmarks in 2011 will be held at the 2010 levels. In 2012, PPACA phases-in blended benchmarks based on a percentage (95%, 100%, 107.5%, or 115%) of a base amount. In 2012, the base amount is to be set at per-capita spending in original Medicare; after 2012, the base amount is either the previous year's base amount increased by the growth in overall Medicare, or per capita spending in original Medicare in that county. The percentage adjustment to the base amount will be determined by the county's per capita FFS spending relative to that of other counties. Counties will be divided into 4 equal groups (or quartiles). The 25% of counties with the highest per capita spending will have a benchmark based on 95% of the base amount. The 25% of counties with the next highest per capita spending in FFS Medicare will have a benchmark based on 100% of the base amount (i.e., 100% of per capita FFS spending in the county). The 25% of counties with the third highest per capita FFS spending will have benchmarks set at 107.5% of the base amount. Counties with the lowest per capita spending in FFS Medicare will have a benchmark based on the 115% of that amount. The phase-in schedule for the new benchmarks varies over two, four, or six years depending on the size of the benchmark reduction, with a longer phase-in schedule for areas where the benchmark decreases by larger amounts. The Secretary will periodically re-rank the counties. If a county's quartile ranking changes, the county will receive a one-year phase-in to the new ranking level. The benchmarks as calculated under the new methodology cannot be greater than what they would have been in the absence of PPACA. The new blended benchmarks does not apply to the Program for All Inclusive Care for the Elderly (PACE plans).[46]

Quality Increases to Benchmarks. PPACA *increases* benchmarks based on plan quality, with higher increases for quality plans in qualifying areas. Starting in 2012, plans with at least a 4-star rating on a 5-star quality rating scale will receive an increase in their benchmark. In 2012, qualifying plans receive a 1.5 percentage point increase in their benchmark; in 2013, the increase is 3.0 percentage points, and starting in 2014, the increase is 5.0 percentage points. The increases are doubled for qualifying plans in a qualifying county. A qualifying county is defined as a county with (1) lower than average per capita spending in original Medicare, (2) 25% or more beneficiaries enrolled in MA, as of December 2009, and (3) a payment rate in 2004 based on the minimum amount applicable to a metropolitan statistical area (i.e., an urban floor rate). New plans or plans with low enrollment, as determined by the Secretary, may also qualify for a benchmark increase. Plans with low enrollment will be deemed to qualify for a quality increase in 2012.[47] Starting in 2013, the Secretary is required to establish a method of determining plan quality for plans with low enrollment. New plans will be deemed to meet the quality requirements, but the percentage increase in their benchmarks will be lower in 2013 and 2014.

Rebates. An MA plan receives a rebate if its bid is below the benchmark. The rebate is equal to a percentage of the difference between the bid and the benchmark. Prior to PPACA, all such plans received a 75% rebate to be used to provide additional benefits not covered under Medicare, reduced cost-sharing, and/or reduced Part B or D premiums. PPACA varies plan rebates based on quality. The highest quality plans (4.5 stars or higher) will receive a 70% rebate if their bid is below the benchmark. Plans with at least 3.5 stars and less than 4.5 stars receive a 65% rebate. Plans with less than 3.5 stars receive a 50% rebate if their bid is below the benchmark. In 2012, plans with low enrollment will be treated as having a 4.5 star rating (with a 70% rebate). Starting in 2012, new plans will be treated as having 3.5 stars. New plans are defined as those that are offered by organizations that have not had a contract as an MA organization in the preceding three years. The change in rebate percentages will be phased in over three years.

Application of Coding Intensity Adjustment. In general, MA plan payments are risk-adjusted to account for the variation in the cost of providing care. Risk adjustment is designed to compensate plans for the increased cost of treating older and sicker beneficiaries, and thus discourage plans from preferential enrollment of healthier individuals. The Deficit Reduction Act of 2005 (P.L. 109-171, DRA) required the Secretary to adjust for patterns of diagnosis coding differences between MA plans and providers under parts A and B of Medicare for plan payments in 2008, 2009, and 2010. PPACA requires the Secretary to conduct further analyses on the differences in coding patterns and adjust for those differences after 2010. Starting in 2014, PPACA specifies minimum coding intensity adjustments. In 2014, the adjustment will be at least the value of the adjustment in 2010 plus 1.3 percentage points; for 2015 to 2018, the adjustment will be not less than the adjustment for the previous year increased by 0.25 percentage points; starting in 2019, the coding intensity adjustment will not be less than 5.7%.

Repeal of Comparative Cost Adjustment Program. Comparative Cost Adjustment is a program required by the Medicare Prescription Drug, Improvement, and Modernization Act of 2003 (P.L. 108-132) to: (1) examine a new MA payment system under which payments to MA plans would be based on a weighted average of plan bids; and (2) introduce possible adjustments (either increases or decreases) to FFS Medicare Part B premiums, based on a comparison of the costs of providing required Medicare benefits to the cost of providing the same benefits in the MA program. PPACA repeals this program. *The CBO score (combined with Section 3209 and Section 1103 of HCERA) is -$30.3 billion for FY2010-FY2014 and -$135.6 billion for FY2010-FY2019.*

Section 1103 of the Reconciliation Act. Savings from Limits on MA Plan Administrative Costs. A Medical Loss Ratio (MLR) identifies the proportion of a plan's premium revenue that the plan devotes to the provision of health care services. The remaining proportion represents the amount spent on managing the plan, including administrative costs, advertising, and profits. Beginning in 2014, PPACA requires plans to have an MLR of less than .85 or remit to the Secretary a payment equal to their total revenue multiplied by the difference between .85 and their MLR. The Secretary is required to restrict enrollment in an MA plan if its MLR was below .85 for three consecutive years and terminate the plan's contract if the plan fails to meet the MLR requirements for five consecutive years. *The CBO score for this section was included in the estimate for Section 3201.*

Sec. 3202. Benefit Protection and Simplification. Under MA, enrollee cost sharing (i.e., coinsurance, copayments, and deductibles) is determined on a plan-by-plan basis. Cost sharing for a particular service may be greater than or less than the cost sharing under original Medicare, and may change from year to year. However, the total value of cost sharing required by an MA plan is constrained by the estimated actuarial value of total cost sharing under original Medicare. Under PPACA, beginning in 2011, MA plans will be prohibited from charging cost sharing that is greater than the cost sharing under original Medicare for certain services including chemotherapy treatment, renal dialysis, skilled nursing care, and services identified by the Secretary.[48] *The CBO score is $0.0 billion for FY2010-FY2014 and $0.0 billion for FY2010-FY2019.*

Sec. 3203. Application of Coding Intensity Adjustment During MA Payment Transition. *This provision was repealed by the Reconciliation Act. A coding intensity adjustment provision was added to Section 3201 and is discussed above.*

Sec. 3204. Simplification of Annual Beneficiary Election Periods. Medicare beneficiaries may enroll in or change their enrollment in MA from November 15 to December 31 each year (the annual, coordinated election period). Changes go into effect January 1st of the next year. During the first 3 months of the year, beneficiaries can enroll in an MA plan, and individuals enrolled in an MA plan can either switch to a different MA plan or return to original Medicare (the continuous open enrollment and disenrollment period). Effective beginning in 2011, PPACA shifts the annual, coordinated election period for MA and Part D to October 15 through December 7. Also beginning in 2011, this provision prohibits beneficiaries from switching MA plans or enrolling in an MA plan from original Medicare after the start of the benefit year. PPACA, however, allows beneficiaries who had enrolled in Medicare Advantage during the annual, coordinated election period to disenroll and return to original Medicare during the first 45-day period of the new benefit year (January 1-February 15), and allows those beneficiaries to enroll in a Part D prescription drug plan. *The CBO score is $0.0 billion for FY2010-FY2014 and $0.0 billion for FY2010-FY2019.*

Sec. 3205. Extension for Specialized MA Plans for Special Needs Individuals. The Medicare Prescription Drug, Improvement, and Modernization Act of 2003 (MMA, P.L. 108-173) established a new type of Medicare Advantage (MA) coordinated care plan focused on individuals with special needs. Special needs plans (SNPs) are allowed to target enrollment to one or more types of special needs individuals including 1) institutionalized; 2) dually eligible; and/or 3) individuals with severe or disabling chronic conditions. This provision extends SNP authority through December 31, 2013. The Secretary is required to establish a frailty payment adjustment, similar to PACE, for fully integrated dual-eligible SNPs. The Secretary only has authority to adjust payments to dual-eligible SNP when those plans have fully integrated Medicare and Medicaid benefits, including long-term care, and met other criteria. Fully integrated dual-eligible SNPs will be exempted from the IME payment phase-out applicable to all MA plans.

In addition, the provision temporarily extends authority through the end of 2012 for SNPs that do not have contracts with state Medicaid programs to continue to operate, but not to expand their service area. The provision requires the Secretary to establish a process to transition SNP beneficiaries that do not qualify as special needs individuals, to fee-for-service Medicare and other MA plans. As part of the transition process, the Secretary will provide for an exception process for beneficiaries who lose Medicaid coverage to reapply for benefits. Beginning in 2012, SNPs will be required to have approval of the National Committee for Quality Assurance in order to serve targeted populations. Periodically, beginning in 2011, the Secretary is required to evaluate, revise, and publish the MA risk adjustment payment methodology to recalibrate payments for higher medical and care coordination costs for specified conditions. *The CBO score (combined with Section 3208) is $0.6 billion for FY2010-FY2014 and $0.7 billion for FY2010-FY2019.*

Sec. 3206. Extension of Reasonable Cost Contracts. Reasonable cost plans are Medicare Advantage (MA) plans that are reimbursed by Medicare for the actual cost of providing services to enrollees. Cost plans were created in the Tax Equity and Fiscal Responsibility Act (TEFRA) of 1982. The Balanced Budget Act of 1997 included a provision to phase-out the reasonable cost contracts, however, the phase-out has been delayed over the years through congressional action. These plans are allowed to operate indefinitely, unless two other plans of the same type (i.e., either 2 local or 2 regional plans) offered by different organizations operate for the entire year in the cost contract's service area. Under prior law, after January 1, 2010, the Secretary could not extend or renew a reasonable cost contract for a service area if (1) during the entire previous year there were either two or more MA regional plans *or* two or more MA local plans in the service area offered by different MA organizations, *and* (2) these regional or local plans meet minimum enrollment requirements. PPACA extends for three years—from January 1, 2010, to January 1, 2013—the length of time reasonable cost plans may continue operating regardless of any other MA plans serving the area. *The CBO score is $0.0 billion for FY2010-FY2014 and $0.0 billion for FY2010-FY2019.*

Sec. 3207. Technical Correction to MA Private Fee-for-Service Plans. MA coordinated care plans are required to meet medical access requirements by forming networks of contracted providers. Prior to 2011, PFFS plans can meet medical access requirements either by establishing payment rates for providers that are not less than rates paid under original Medicare or by developing contracts and agreements with a sufficient number and range of providers within a category to provide covered services under the terms of the plan. Starting in 2011, PFFS plans sponsored by employers or unions are required to establish contracted networks of providers to meet access requirements. Non-employer sponsored MA PFFS plans are required to establish contracted networks of providers in "network areas" defined as areas having at least two plans with networks (such as health maintenance organizations [HMOs], provider sponsored organizations [PSOs], or local preferred provider organizations [PPOs]). In areas without at least two network-based plans, the non-employer

PFFS plans retain the ability to establish access requirements through establishing payment rates that are not less than those under original Medicare.

PPACA allows the Secretary to grant employer-based PFFS plans with enrollment as of October 1, 2009, a waiver from the network requirements in a manner similar to the Secretary's authority to waive or modify other MA requirements for employer-based coordinated care plans as specified in a 2008 service area extension waiver policy, as modified in an April 11, 2008 CMS memo entitled "2009 Employer Group Waiver-Modification of the 2008 Service Area Extension Waiver Granted to Certain MA Local Coordinated Care Plans." *The CBO score is $0.0 billion for FY2010-FY2014 and $0.1 billion for FY2010-FY2019.*

Sec. 3208. Making Senior Housing Facility Demonstration Permanent. In general, MA plans are required to serve an area no smaller than a county, which prevents plans from targeting smaller areas of healthier, low-cost enrollees. However, it is possible for an MA plan to receive a waiver of this requirement to be able to restrict enrollment to residents of a retirement community. Effective January 1, 2010, PPACA requires the Secretary to establish a new type of MA plan called an MA Senior Housing Facility Plan, which is to be allowed to limit its service area to a senior housing facility within a geographic area. An MA Senior Housing Facility Plan is to be an MA plan that serves beneficiaries who reside in a continuing care retirement community, has a sufficient number of on-site primary care providers as determined by the Secretary, supplies transportation benefits to other providers, and were in existence under a demonstration for at least one year. *The CBO score for this section was included in the estimate for Section 3205.*

Sec. 3209. Authority to Deny Plan Bids. In general, the Secretary has the authority to negotiate bids submitted by MA plans similar to the authority of the Director of the Office of Personnel Management with respect to negotiations with plans participating in the Federal Employees Health Benefits Program. The Secretary may only accept a bid after determining that it is supported actuarially and that it reasonably and equitably reflects the revenue requirements of benefits provided under the plan. The Secretary's authority to negotiate with plans does not apply to Private Fee-for-Service (PFFS) MA plans. Effective January 1, 2011, PPACA clarifies that the Secretary is not required to accept any or every bid submitted by an MA plan or Part D prescription drug plan. *The CBO score for this section was included in the estimate for Section 3201.*

Sec. 3210. Development of New Standards for Certain Medigap Plans. Many Medicare beneficiaries have individually purchased health insurance policies, commonly referred to as "Medigap" policies. Beneficiaries with Medigap insurance typically have coverage for Medicare's deductibles and coinsurance; they may also have coverage for some items and services not covered by Medicare. Individuals generally select from one of a set of standardized plans (Plan "A" through Plan "L", though not all plans are offered in all states). The law incorporates by reference, as part of the statutory requirements, certain minimum standards established by the National Association of Insurance Commissioners (NAIC) and provides for modification where appropriate to reflect program changes. PPACA requests that NAIC create new model plans for C and F that include nominal cost sharing to encourage the use of appropriate Part B physician services. The nominal cost sharing is to be based on evidence either published or from integrated delivery systems. The revisions are to be consistent with rules applicable to changes in NAIC Model Regulations. The new models C and F are to be available in 2015. *The CBO score is $0.0 billion for FY2010-FY2014 and -$0.1 billion for FY2010-FY2019.*

Sec. 10327(c). Elimination of MA Regional Plan Stabilization Fund. MMA created the MA Regional Program and established the MA Regional Plan Stabilization Fund to encourage plans to enter into and/or remain in the MA Regional Program. The fund was originally set at $10 billion with additional money added to the fund from savings in the bidding process. Funds were to be available from 2007 through the end of 2013. Subsequent legislation decreased the amount of funds available and delayed their availability. Most recently, MIPPA reduced the initial funding of the program to one dollar. Money from the regional plan bidding process continued to flow into the Fund, but availability had been delayed until 2014. PPACA eliminates the Fund and transfers amounts in the Fund to the Part B Trust Fund. *The CBO score is -$0.1 billion for FY2010-FY2014 and -$0.2 billion for FY2010-FY2019.*

Subtitle D—Medicare Part D Improvements for Prescription Drug Plans and MA-PD Plans

Sec. 3301 as modified by Sec. 1101 of the Reconciliation Act. Medicare Coverage Gap Discount Program for Brand-Name Drugs and Closing the Medicare Prescription Drug "Donut Hole."

Medicare law sets out a defined standard benefit structure under the Part D prescription drug benefit that includes a gap in coverage, commonly referred to as the "doughnut hole." In 2010, the standard benefit includes a $310 deductible and a 25% coinsurance until the enrollee reaches $2,830 in total covered drug spending (Medicare and beneficiary spending combined). After this initial coverage limit is reached, the enrollee is responsible for the full cost of the drugs until total costs hit the catastrophic threshold, $6,440 in 2010. In general, in 2010, Part D enrollees who do not receive assistance in the form of the Part D low-income subsidy would be responsible for a total of $4,550 in out-of-pocket costs before reaching the catastrophic phase ($310 deductible, $630 in co-insurance in the initial coverage phase, and $3,610 in the coverage gap).[49]

This provision incorporates a voluntary agreement with the Pharmaceutical Research and Manufacturers of America (PhRMA) to provide discounts of 50% for brand-name drugs used by Part D enrollees in the Part D coverage gap. Manufacturers of prescription drugs will be required to enter into agreements with Medicare Part D drug plan sponsors to provide discounts on drugs provided to plan enrollees in the coverage gap period beginning January 1, 2011. The amount of the discount, in addition to the amount actually paid by the enrollee, will count toward costs incurred by the plan enrollee. Plan enrollees receiving the low-income subsidy or enrolled in an employee–sponsored retiree drug plan will not be eligible for the discount. Drugs sold and marketed in the U.S. by a manufacturer will not be covered under Part D unless the manufacturer agrees to participate in the discount program. The provision also requires the Secretary to contract with a third party entity (or entities) to administer the drug discount program and to establish performance requirements and data standards for the third-party contractor(s).

Section 1101 of the Reconciliation Act added provisions to close the coverage gap by 2020 and to provide for an immediate reduction in costs for beneficiaries who enter the coverage gap in 2010. Specifically, in 2010, Medicare Part D enrollees who enter the coverage gap will receive a rebate of $250. Additionally, the Reconciliation Act reduces beneficiary cost sharing for *brand-name drugs* from 100% in 2010 (minus the $250 rebate) to 25% by 2020. In 2011 and 2012, per the manufacturer discount provision in PPACA, beneficiary cost-sharing will be reduced to 50% of the price of the drug. In 2013 and beyond, the Medicare program will cover additional costs beyond the 50% discount to further reduce cost-sharing; in total, beneficiary cost-sharing for brand-name drugs during the coverage gap will be 47.5% in 2013 and 2014, 45% in 2015 and 2016, 40% in 2017, 35% in 2018, 30% in 2019, and 25% in 2020 and beyond (in 2020, the manufacturer discounts account for 50% of the reduction and the Medicare Part D program pays the remaining 25%). For *generic drugs*, which are not subject the required 50% discount, beneficiary cost-sharing in the coverage gap will be reduced to 93% in 2011; in 2012 and for each succeeding year, the percentage will decrease by an additional 7%,[50] until 2020 when beneficiaries' cost-sharing for generic drugs will equal 25% (in 2020, the Medicare Part D program will pay 75% of the cost of generic drugs).

The Reconciliation Act also makes several modifications to the methodology used to determine updates to the total out-of-pocket expenditure amounts for years 2014 through 2019. In general, these changes will reduce the rate of growth in the total amount that Part D enrollees would need to spend before reaching the catastrophic threshold for these years.[51] *The CBO score is +$9.2 billion for FY2010-FY2014 and +$42.6 billion for FY2010-FY2019.*[52]

Sec. 3302. Improvement in Determination of Part D Low-Income Benchmark Premium. The federal government pays up to 100% of the Part D premiums for low-income subsidy (LIS) beneficiaries who are enrolled in "benchmark" plans. A Part D plan qualifies as a benchmark plan if it offers basic Part D coverage with premiums equal to or lower than the regional low-income premium subsidy amount. MA plans offering prescription drug coverage submit a separate bid for the Part D portion. Payment for the portion of the premium attributable to basic prescription drug benefits is calculated in the same way as that for stand-alone PDPs, however an MA plan may choose to apply some of its Part C rebate payments to lower the Part D premium. If an MA plan uses rebate payments to reduce its Part D premium, this reduced amount is factored into the calculation of the regional low-income benchmark. This has the effect of lowering the benchmark and potentially of reducing the number of plans that qualify as low-income plans. MedPAC has noted that the number of plans that qualify as low-income benchmark plans has been decreasing in recent years, resulting in fewer options for LIS enrollees. This provision excludes the Medicare Advantage rebate amounts from the MA-PDP premium bids when calculating the low-income regional benchmark. This provision will be effective starting in the 2011 plan year. *The CBO score is +$0.3 billion for FY2010-FY2014 and +$0.7 billion for FY2010-FY2019.*

Sec. 3303. Voluntary De Minimus Policy for Subsidy Eligible Individuals Under Prescription Drug Plans and MA-PD Plans. To help maintain plans that wish to serve LIS beneficiaries at fully subsidized or $0 premiums, this provision authorizes a policy, beginning in 2011, through which plans that bid a nominal amount above the regional low-income subsidy (LIS) benchmark amount could choose to absorb the cost of the small difference between their bid and the LIS benchmark in order to qualify as a LIS-eligible plan. The Secretary has discretion to auto-enroll LIS beneficiaries into these plans in order to maintain adequate LIS plan choices. The de minimus threshold amount will be established by the Secretary. *The CBO score is +$0.1 billion for FY2010-FY2014 and +$0.4 billion for FY2010-FY2019.*

Sec. 3304. Special Rule for Widows and Widowers Regarding Eligibility for Low-Income Assistance. To qualify for financial assistance under the Part D low-income subsidy (LIS) program, Medicare beneficiaries must have resources no greater than the income and resource limits established by the Medicare Prescription Drug, Improvement, and Modernization Act of 2003 (MMA, P.L. 108-173). Each year, the Secretary conducts a redeeming process to determine whether those who automatically qualified for the full subsidy in a given year continue to meet the criteria for eligibility in the following year. For those who have qualified for the full or partial subsidy through the application process, the agency that made the determination decision (SSA or an individual state) is responsible for monitoring a recipient's eligibility. For example, for cases in which eligibility has been established through an application with SSA, a report of a subsidy-changing event, such as marriage, divorce, or death of a spouse, will trigger a redetermination of subsidy eligibility during the calendar year. This can result in changes to the individual's deductible, premium and cost sharing subsidy, or even termination of his or her LIS eligibility status. In the case of the death of a spouse, it is possible that the surviving spouse, as the sole owner of the previously combined resources, may exceed the resource limit for an individual and may no longer qualify for the LIS program.

This provision requires that, beginning in 2011, the surviving spouse of an LIS-eligible couple undergo a redetermination of his or her eligibility status no earlier than one year from the next redetermination that would have occurred after the death of a spouse. Subsequently, the LIS widow/widower is to be determined or redetermined, as appropriate, for LIS on the same basis as other LIS-eligible beneficiaries. *The CBO score is +$0.1 billion for FY2010-FY2014 and +$0.2 billion for FY2010-FY2019.*

Sec. 3305. Improved Information for Subsidy Eligible Individuals Reassigned to Prescription Drug Plans and MA-PD Plans. According to the Medicare Prescription Drug, Improvement, and Modernization Act of 2003 (MMA, P.L. 108-173), low-income subsidy (LIS) beneficiaries who are enrolled in plans with premiums below the low-income regional benchmark amount receive assistance with premiums and cost sharing. Those who are enrolled in LIS-eligible plans whose plan bids exceed the regional benchmark amount for the next benefit year are randomly reassigned by the Secretary of HHS to new plans whose bids are at or below the regional benchmark amount in order to ensure that these beneficiaries continue to receive a subsidy of plan premiums. It is possible that the new plan's exceptions, appeals and grievance mechanisms could differ from the old plan and that some covered drug(s) a beneficiary is currently taking would not be covered by the new plan.

In the case of an LIS beneficiary who has been reassigned to another LIS plan, the provision requires the Secretary, beginning in 2011, to transmit within 30 days of the reassignment information to the beneficiary about formulary differences between the former plan and the new plan with respect to the beneficiary's drug regimen, as well as a description of the beneficiary's rights to request a coverage determination, exception or reconsideration, or resolve a grievance. *The CBO score is $0.0 billion for FY2010-FY2014 and $0.0 billion for FY2010-FY2019.*

Sec. 3306. Funding Outreach and Assistance for Low-Income Programs. Section 119 of the Medicare Improvements for Patients and Providers Act of 2008 (MIPPA, P.L. 110-275) provided $25 million for fiscal years 2008 and 2009 for beneficiary outreach and education activities related to low-income programs related to the Medicare through State Health Insurance Counseling and Assistance Programs (SHIPs), Area Agencies on Aging (AAAs), Aging and Disability Resource Centers (ADRCs), and the Administration on Aging (AoA). This provision extends MIPPA Section 119 and provides an additional $45 million for outreach and education activities related to Medicare low-income assistance programs, including the Part D low-income subsidy (LIS) program and the Medicare Savings Program (MSP). Funds are to be allocated to SHIPs, AAAs, ADRCs, and the National Center for Benefits Outreach and Enrollment in the same proportion as under MIPPA and will be available for obligation through 2012. The Secretary was also provided the authority to enlist the support of these entities to conduct outreach activities aimed at preventing disease and promoting wellness as an additional use of these funds. *The CBO score is $0.0 billion for FY2010-FY2014 and $0.0 billion for FY2010-FY2019.*

Sec. 3307. Improving Formulary Requirements for Prescription Drug Plans and MA-PD Plans with Respect to Certain Categories or Classes of Drugs. The Medicare Prescription Drug, Improvement, and Modernization Act of 2003 (MMA, P.L. 108-173) requires Part D plans to operate formularies that cover drugs within each therapeutic category and class of covered Part D drugs, although not necessarily all drugs within such categories and classes. The Secretary of HHS published a regulation (42 CFR Section 423.120) that requires Part D plans to have at least two drugs within each therapeutic category and class. However, through sub-regulatory guidance, the Secretary protected access to certain classes of drugs by requiring Part D plans to cover all, or substantially all, of the drugs in the following six drug classes: immunosuppressant, antidepressant, antipsychotic, anticonvulsant, antiretroviral, and anti-neoplastic. Section 176 of the Medicare Improvements for Patients and Providers Act of 2008 (MIPPA, P.L. 110-275) codified that, beginning in plan year 2010, the Secretary would identify the classes and categories of drugs that should be protected, or covered entirely by Part D plans, to ensure that beneficiaries have access to certain therapies and to a wide variety of therapy options for certain conditions and established certain criteria the Secretary would use to identify such drugs.

This provision of PPACA gives the Secretary authority to identify classes of clinical concern as defined by the Secretary and PDP sponsors will be required to include all drugs in these classes in their formularies. The provision also codifies the current six classes of clinical concern as they are currently specified through sub-regulatory guidance until the Secretary issues a rule regarding classes of clinical concern to be protected on plan formularies. The provision also removes the criteria specified in Section 176 of MIPPA that would have been used by the Secretary to identify protected classes of drugs. The provision will be effective starting the 2011 plan year. *The CBO score is $0.0 billion for FY2010-FY2014 and $0.0 billion for FY2010-FY2019.*

Sec. 3308. Reducing Part D Premium Subsidy for High-Income Beneficiaries. Beginning in 2007, as required by the MMA, high-income beneficiaries are required to pay higher premiums for Part B benefits. Beneficiaries with modified adjusted gross income that exceeds a threshold amount are charged additional premiums based on a sliding scale that ranges from 35% to 80% of the value of Part B. In 2010, threshold levels start at $85,000 for an individual tax return and $170,000 for a joint return (based on 2008 returns). The threshold amounts are specified in the law, and are adjusted annually for inflation using the Consumer Price Index (CPI). The income thresholds are tied to specific premium shares. Beneficiary premiums under Part D are not subject to income thresholds or means testing. This provision requires Part D enrollees who exceed certain income thresholds to pay higher premiums. The income thresholds will be set in a similar manner to those under Part B. The provision will also inflate the income thresholds by the CPI, except for the period between 2010 and 2019 when the income thresholds would not be updated. In addition, the provision expands the current authority for IRS to disclose income information to SSA for purposes of adjusting the Part B subsidy to include the Part D subsidy adjustments. *The CBO score is -$2.4 billion for FY2010-FY2014 and -$10.7 billion for FY2010-FY2019.*

Sec. 3309. Elimination of Cost Sharing for Certain Dual Eligible Individuals. Cost-sharing subsides for LIS enrollees are linked to the standard Part D prescription drug coverage. Full-subsidy eligibles have no deductible, minimal cost sharing during the initial coverage period and coverage gap, and no cost-sharing over the catastrophic threshold. Full-benefit dual eligibles who are residents of medical institutions or nursing facilities have no cost-sharing. This provision will eliminate cost sharing for drugs dispensed to beneficiaries receiving care under a home and community based waiver who would otherwise require institutional care. This provision is effective on a date specified by the Secretary, but no earlier than January 1, 2012. *The CBO score is +$0.3 billion for FY2010-FY2014 and +$1.1 billion for FY2010-FY2019.*

Sec. 3310. Reducing Wasteful Dispensing of Outpatient Prescription Drugs in Long-Term Care Facilities Under Prescription Drug Plans and MA-PD Plans. Part D plans are required to offer a contract to any pharmacy willing to participate in its long-term care (LTC) pharmacy network so long as the pharmacy is capable of meeting certain minimum performance and service criteria and any other standard terms and conditions established by the plan for its network pharmacies. Each LTC facility selects at least one eligible LTC pharmacy to provide Medicare drug benefits to its residents. Plan formularies must be structured so that they meet the needs of long-term care residents and provide coverage for all medically necessary medications at all levels of care. Both physician prescribing patterns and pharmacy benefit manager (PBM) payment practices result in prescriptions commonly being dispensed in 30- or 90-day quantities. In situations when the full amount dispensed is not utilized by the patient, for example. due to discharge, death, adverse reactions, the remaining medication may become waste. This provision will require Part D sponsors, starting January 1, 2012, to employ utilization management techniques, determined by the Secretary in consultation with relevant stakeholders, to reduce the quantity dispensed per fill when dispensing medications to beneficiaries who reside in long-term care facilities in order to reduce waste associated with 30-day fills. These techniques could include such things as weekly, daily, or automated dose dispensing. *The CBO score is -$1.0 billion for FY2010-FY2014 and -$5.7 billion for FY2010-FY2019.*

Sec. 3311. Improved Medicare Prescription Drug Plan and MA-PD Complaint System. Part D and Medicare Advantage (MA) related complaints are tracked and resolved through a centralized complaints system within the Centers for Medicare & Medicaid Services (CMS), while complaints submitted directly to plan sponsors (grievances) are tracked and resolved by each plan sponsor using its own system. CMS maintains a central repository of MA and Part D- related complaints received by its Regional Offices, Central Office, or through 1-800- MEDICARE. This provision requires the Secretary to develop and maintain a system, which is widely known and easy to use, to handle complaints regarding MA and Part D plans or their sponsors. The system is to have the ability to report and initiate appropriate interventions and monitoring based on substantial complaints and to guide quality improvement. A plan complaint is defined as a complaint that is received (including by telephone, letter, e-mail, or any other means) by the Secretary (including by a regional office, the Medicare Beneficiary Ombudsman, a sub-contractor, a carrier, a fiscal intermediary, or a Medicare Administrative Contractor). The Secretary is required to develop a model electronic complaint form to be used for reporting complaints under the system that would be displayed on the Medicare.gov and Medicare Beneficiary Ombudsman websites. The Secretary is also required to conduct annual reports of the complaint system that would include an analysis of the numbers and types of complaints reported under the system; geographic variations in the complaints; the timeliness of agency or plan responses to the complaints; and the resolution of the complaints. *The CBO score is $0.0 billion for FY2010-FY2014 and $0.0 billion for FY2010-FY2019.*

Sec. 3312. Uniform Exceptions and Appeals Process for Prescription Drug Plans and MA-PD Plans. Section 1852(g) of the Social Security Act outlines general requirements regarding Medicare Advantage exceptions and appeals processes. The Part D program adapted many of the existing rules for appeals that apply to Medicare Advantage program. The coverage and determination and appeals processes may vary among MA and Part D plans as long as these general requirements are met. This provision will require a prescription drug plan sponsor or a MA organization offering MA-PD plans to use a single, uniform exceptions and appeals process with respect to the determination of prescription drug coverage for an enrollee under the plan and to provide instant access to this process through a toll-free telephone number and an Internet website. This provision will apply to exceptions and appeals made on or after January 1, 2012. *The CBO score is $0.0 billion for FY2010-FY2014 and $0.0 billion for FY2010-FY2019.*

Sec. 3313. Office of the Inspector General Studies and Reports. According to Section 1860D-14 of the SSA, full-benefit dual-eligible individuals who have not elected a Part D plan are to be auto-enrolled into one by CMS. Because plans vary in the formularies they offer, some dual eligibles could find that they have been auto-enrolled in a plan that may not best meet their needs. Additionally, when the Medicare prescription drug program was created, it was expected that drug plan sponsors would negotiate with drug manufacturers to obtain price concessions on drugs covered under Part D, and thus reduce total costs to the government and to beneficiaries. Some studies have suggested that Part D plans are not obtaining rebates equivalent to those required under Medicaid.

PPACA requires the Office of Inspector General of HHS (OIG) to report annually, beginning July 1, 2011, on the extent to which formularies used by prescription drug plans and MA-PD plans under Part D include drugs commonly used by full-benefit dual eligible individuals. OIG is also required to complete a study by October 1, 2011, that compares covered prescription drug prices paid under the Medicare Part D program to those negotiated by state Medicaid plans for the top 200 drugs determined by both volume and expenditures including all rebates and discounts received by the Medicaid and Part D plans. The report is not to disclose information that is deemed proprietary or likely to negatively impact a Medicaid program or Part D plans' ability to negotiate drug prices. *The CBO score is $0.0 billion for FY2010-FY2014 and $0.0 billion for FY2010-FY2019.*

Sec. 3314. Including Costs Incurred By AIDS Drug Assistance Programs And Indian Health Service In Providing Prescription Drugs Toward The Annual Out Of Pocket Threshold Under Part D. Under a standard Medicare Part D plan design, beneficiaries must incur a certain level of out-of-pocket costs ($4,550 in 2010) before catastrophic protection begins. These include costs that are incurred for the deductible, cost-sharing, or benefits not paid because they fall in the coverage gap. Generally, costs are counted as incurred, and thus treated as true out-of-pocket (true out-of-pocket) costs only if they are paid by the individual (or by another family member on behalf of the individual), paid on behalf of a low-income individual under the subsidy provisions, or paid under a State Pharmaceutical Assistance Program. Additional payments that do not count toward TrOOP include Part D premiums and coverage by other insurance, including group health plans, workers' compensation, Part D plans' supplemental or enhanced benefits, or other third parties. This provision will allow costs paid by the Indian Health Service or under an AIDS Drug Assistance Program to count toward the out-of-pocket threshold for costs incurred on or after January 1, 2011. *The CBO score is +$0.2 billion for FY2010-FY2014 and +$0.6 billion for FY2010-FY2019.*

Sec. 3315. Immediate Reduction in Coverage Gap in 2010 (*repealed by Section 1101 of the Reconciliation Act*).

Sec. 10328. Improvement in Part D Medication Therapy Management (MTM) Programs. Section 1860-D-4(c) of the SSA requires Part D sponsors to incorporate a Medication Therapy Management Program (MTM) into their plan benefit structures. An MTM program is a program of drug therapy management that may be furnished by a pharmacist and is designed to assure, with respect to targeted beneficiaries, that covered Part D drugs are appropriately used to optimize therapeutic outcomes through improved medication use and to reduce the risk of adverse events. Targeted individuals are those who have multiple chronic diseases, are taking multiple covered part D drugs, and are identified to likely incur annual costs for covered Part D drugs that exceed a level specified by the Secretary. The MTM program may include elements that promote enrollee understanding of the appropriate use of medication and increased adherence with medication regimes, and must be developed in cooperation with licensed and practicing pharmacists and physicians. This provision amends Section 1860D-4(c) to require Part D sponsors to include in their MTM programs an annual comprehensive medication review furnished in person or using telehealth technologies by a licensed pharmacist or other qualified provider, and follow-up interventions as warranted based on the findings of the annual review or the targeted medication enrollment starting in plan years beginning on or after the date that is 2 years after the date of enactment. Additionally, the plan sponsor will be required to have in place a process to assess on a quarterly basis the medication use of individuals who are at risk but not enrolled in the MTM program, including individuals who have experienced a transition in care. The plan sponsor will also be required to have in place a process to automatically enroll targeted beneficiaries in the MTM program and permit such beneficiaries to opt out of enrollment in the program. The Secretary of HHS has been given authority to modify or broaden requirements for MTM programs and to study new MTM models through the Center for Medicare and Medicaid Innovation (as added by Section 3021). *The CBO score is $0.0 billion for FY2010-FY2014 and $0.0 billion for FY2010-FY2019.*

Subtitle E—Ensuring Medicare Sustainability

Sec. 3401 as modified by Sec. 10319 of PPACA, and Sec. 1105 of the Reconciliation Act. Revision of Certain Market Basket Updates and Incorporation of Productivity Improvements into Market Basket Updates That Do Not Already Incorporate Such Improvements. Most fee-for-service Medicare providers receive predetermined payment amounts established under different, unique prospective payment systems. Each year, the base payment amounts in the different Medicare payment systems are increased by an update factor to reflect the increase in the unit costs associated with providing health care services. Generally, Medicare's annual updates are linked to either: (1) projected changes in specific market basket (MB) indices which are designed to measure the change in the price of goods and services (such as labor and equipment) that are purchased by the provider and intended to reflect the effect of inflation on providers' costs per service; or (2) the Consumer Price Index for All Urban Consumers (CPI-U). Generally, PPACA provides for updates based on the MB or CPI minus full productivity estimates for all Parts A and B providers and suppliers who are subject to a MB or CPI update. The productivity offset is to equal the percentage change in the 10-year moving average of annual economy-wide private nonfarm business multi-factor productivity. The estimate used will be that published before the promulgation of the regulation establishing increases in the Medicare rates for the year or period.

Specifically, this provision will implement a full productivity adjustment for inpatient hospital services, inpatient rehabilitation, long-term care hospital services, skilled nursing facilities and hospices beginning October 1, 2012, for inpatient psychiatric facilities beginning July 1, 2012, for hospital outpatient departments beginning January 1, 2012, and for home health providers beginning in October 1, 2014. For providers paid through the clinical laboratory test fee schedule, the proposal will replace the scheduled 0.5% payment reduction for calendar years 2011 through 2013 with a full productivity adjustment for calendar year (CY) 2011 and subsequent years. Dialysis providers will be subject to the productivity adjustment starting in CY2012; the productivity adjustments for other Part B providers will begin in CY2011. Except where noted below, the application of the update adjustments may result in a negative factor and a basis of payment that would be lower than in the preceding year. The update factors for Medicare providers and suppliers will be subject to the following adjustments:

Acute care hospitals, long-term care hospitals, inpatient rehabilitation facilities, inpatient psychiatric facilities, and outpatient hospitals: Aside from the productivity factors mentioned earlier, the MB update for acute care inpatient (IPPS) services and inpatient rehabilitation facilities (IRFs) will be reduced 0.25 percentage points starting in FY2010, effective for discharges starting April 1, 2010) and FY2011; 0.1 percentage points in FY2012 and FY2013; 0.3 percentage points in FY2014; 0.2 percentage points in FY2015 and FY2016; and 0.75 percentage points in FY2017 though FY2019. These same reductions also apply to the update for long-term care hospitals except that a larger reduction of 0.5 percentage points will apply starting October 1, 2010 (RY2010). The MB update for the hospital outpatient prospective system will be reduced 0.25 percentage points in CY2010 and CY2011 and by 0.1 percentage points in CY2012 and CY2013. 0.3 percentage points in CY2014; 0.2 percentage points in CY2015 and CY2016; and 0.75 percentage points in CY2017 though CY2019. *Skilled nursing facilities:* The SNF MB update will be subject to the productivity factor adjustment beginning in FY2012. *Home health agencies:* Aside from the productivity factor adjustment beginning in 2015, the MB update for home health services will be reduced by 1.0 percentage point in CY2011, CY2012, and CY2013. *Hospice care:* The hospice MB update will be subject to the productivity factor adjustment beginning in FY2013. Aside from the productivity factor adjustment, the MB update will be reduced by 0.3 percentage points in FY2013. For each of the fiscal years from FY2014 through FY2019, a 0.3 percentage point reduction to the MB will be contingent upon the level of the insured population relative to the projection of insured population for the year preceding enactment. Specifically, only if the level of non-elderly insured population is 5 or fewer percentage points above the projections would the MB update be reduced by 0.3 percentage points. *Dialysis:* The ESRD MB will no longer be subject to a 1 percentage point reduction beginning in 2012, but will be subject to the productivity factor adjustments starting in CY2012. *Ambulance services:* The productivity adjustment factor will be applied to the CPI-U used to increase the ambulance fee schedule starting in CY2011. *Ambulatory surgical services:* The productivity adjustment factor will be applied to the CPI-U used to update payments for ambulatory surgical services starting in CY2011. *Laboratory services:* The existing 0.5 percentage point reduction to the CPI-U update to the fee schedule in CY2009 and CY2010 will be retained. A 1.75 percentage point reduction to the update in CY2011 through CY2015 will be established; this reduction may result in a negative update. The productivity adjustment factor will be applied to the CPI-U starting in CY2011, but in the application of the adjustment will not be able to reduce the increase to less than zero. *Certain durable medical equipment:* The productivity adjustment factor will be applied to the CPI-U used to increase the fee schedules for certain durable medical equipment (DME) beginning in CY2011. Certain DME would have received a payment increase of CPI-U plus 2 percentage points in CY2014. The 2 percentage point increase was eliminated. *Prosthetic devices, orthotics, and prosthetics:* The productivity adjustment factor will be applied to the CPI-U update for the applicable fee schedule for this DME category starting in CY2011. *Other items:* The productivity adjustment factor will be applied to the CPI-U update for this DME category starting in CY2011. (See Appendix B for timeline of update reductions including productivity adjustments.) *The CBO score is -$23.7 billion for FY2010-FY2014 and -$156.6 billion for FY2010-FY2019.*[53]

Sec. 3402. Temporary Adjustment to the Calculation of Part B Premiums. Medicare Part B finances coverage for physicians' and other outpatient services, in part, through premiums paid by beneficiaries who enroll in the voluntary program. Before January 2007, the Part B premium was set at 25% of the program's costs per aged enrollee (enrollees who were age 65 or older) and was applied universally to all enrollees. Since then, under a provision of the Medicare Modernization Act, approximately 1.7 million higher-income beneficiaries have faced progressively greater shares of those costs—35 percent, 50 percent, 65 percent, or 80 percent, depending on income. The income categories that those shares apply to are based on enrollees' modified adjusted gross income. In 2010, the income thresholds for those premium shares are \$85,000, \$107,000, \$160,000, and \$214,000, respectively. (For married couples, the corresponding income thresholds are twice those values.) The income thresholds rise each year with changes in the consumer price index. The provision will freeze the current income thresholds for the period of 2011 through 2019 at the 2010 levels. *The CBO score is -\$7.5 billion for FY2010-FY2014 and is -\$25.0 billion for FY2010-FY2019.*

Sec. 3403 as modified by Sec. 10320. Independent Payment Advisory Board.[54] This provision establishes an Independent Payment Advisory Board to develop and submit detailed proposals to Congress and the President to reduce Medicare spending. The Board is to consist of 15 members with expertise in health care financing, delivery, and organization. All members are to be appointed by the President and confirmed by the Senate. Proposals are to primarily focus on payments to MA and PDP plans and reimbursement rates for certain providers. The Board will be prohibited from developing proposals related to Medicare benefits, eligibility, or financing. Proposals, which will only be required in certain years, will have to meet specific savings targets. Recommendations made by the Board automatically go into effect unless Congress enacts specific legislation to prevent their implementation. The first year the Board's proposals can take effect is 2015.

Membership and Structure. The Board is to be composed of 15 members, appointed by the President with the advice and consent of the Senate. Members of the Board will serve six-year, staggered terms. Members may not serve more than 2 full consecutive terms. The Senate Majority Leader, the Speaker of the House, the Senate Minority Leader, and the House Minority Leader will each present three recommendations for appointees to the President. The President, with the advice and consent of the Senate, is required to appoint a Chair for the Board. The Board will elect a Vice Chairman. Members can only be removed by the President for neglect of duty or malfeasance in office. In addition to the 15 members of the Board, the Secretary of Health and Human Services (HHS), the Administrator of the Center for Medicare and Medicaid Services (CMS), and the Administrator of the Health Resources and Services Administration (HRSA) will serve as ex-officio, non-voting members of the Board.

Qualifications for membership are similar to the qualifications required for members of the Medicare Payment Advisory Board (MedPAC). Individuals involved in the delivery or management of health care services cannot constitute a majority of the Board. In addition to these qualifications, the President is required to establish a system for publicly disclosing any financial or other conflicts of interests relating to members. Individuals that engage in any other business, vocation, or employment cannot serve as appointed members of the Board.

Members will be considered officers in the executive branch for purposes of applying Title I of the Ethics in Government Act of 1978. After serving on the Board, former members will be barred from lobbying the Board and other relevant executive branch departments and agencies and relevant congressional committees for one year.

The Chair will be responsible for exercising all of the Board's executive and administrative functions, including those related to the appointment and supervision of employees and the use of funds. All requests for discretionary appropriations to fund the Board's activities must be approved by a majority vote.

Requirements for Proposal Submission. The provision requires that the Board submit proposals to the President for years in which the projected rate of growth in Medicare spending per beneficiary exceeds a target growth rate. Determinations of the projected and target growth rates are to be made by the CMS Office of the Actuary (OACT) beginning in 2013.[55] The Board is required to submit its first proposal to the President by January 15, 2014, for implementation in 2015. If the Board fails to submit a proposal to the President by January 15, the Secretary will be required to submit a contingent proposal to Congress meeting the same requirements by January 25.

For years 2014 through 2017, the Board will be required to submit proposals for years in which the projected rate of growth in Medicare spending per beneficiary exceeds the average of the projected percentage increase in the Consumer Price Index for All Urban Consumers (CPI) and the Consumer Price Index for Medical Care (CPI-M). Beginning in 2018, proposals will only be required for years in which the projected rate of growth in Medicare spending exceeds the Gross Domestic Product (GDP) plus 1.0%. Recommendations proposed by the Board are required to reduce Medicare spending by the lesser of 0.5 percentage points in 2015, 1.0 percentage points in 2016, 1.25 percentage points in 2017, 1.5 percentage points in 2018, and the amount by which the rate of growth in Medicare spending exceeds the target growth rate. Proposals cannot increase Medicare spending over a 10-year period.

Scope of Proposals. The provision lays out a number of specific fiscal and policy criteria which the Board will be required to meet in making its recommendations. When developing and submitting proposals, the Board is required, to the extent feasible, to (1) prioritize recommendations that would extend Medicare solvency and target reductions to sources of excess cost growth; (2) include only those recommendations that improve the health care delivery system, including the promotion of integrated care, care coordination, prevention and wellness and quality improvement and protect beneficiary access to care, including in rural and frontier areas; (3) consider the effects of changes in provider and supplier payments on beneficiaries; consider the effects of proposals on any provider who has, or is projected to have, negative profit margins or payment updates; (4) consider the unique needs of individuals dually eligible for Medicare and Medicaid, and (5) include recommendations for administrative funding to carry out its recommendations.

As appropriate, each proposal is required to include recommendations that would reduce spending in Medicare Parts C and D. Reductions could be obtained by reducing Medicare payments for administrative expenses to MA and PDP plans, denying or removing high bids for drug coverage from the calculation of the monthly bid amount for Part D plans, and reducing performance bonuses for MA plans. Recommendations may not target the base beneficiary premium percentage or the full premium subsidy for Part D plans.

The Board is prohibited from making recommendations that would ration care, raise revenues, increase beneficiary premiums, increase beneficiary cost-sharing, restrict benefits, or modify eligibility. Additionally, proposals submitted before December 2018 for implementation in 2020, cannot include recommendations that would reduce payments to providers and suppliers scheduled to receive a reduction in their payment updates in excess of a reduction due to productivity.

Presidential Review. At the beginning of the year following the determination by the Secretary, the Advisory Board is to submit its recommendations to the President who is to, in turn, immediately submit them to Congress. The provision dictates certain information which must accompany the Advisory Board's submission, including a requirement for legislative language implementing the recommendations.

Congressional Consideration. Section 3403 directs the Secretary to automatically implement the Board's recommendations unless Congress, by August 15 of the year in which the recommendations are submitted, enacts legislation superseding the Board's proposal. The provision establishes special "fast track" parliamentary procedures governing congressional consideration of legislation implementing the Board's recommendations. These fast track procedures differ from the normal parliamentary mechanisms used by the chambers to consider most legislation and are designed to ensure that Congress, should it choose to do so, can act quickly on the proposal put forth by the Advisory Board.

The fast track procedures established by the provision mandate the introduction of the Board's legislative proposal by the House and Senate majority leaders "by request" on the day it is submitted to Congress. When introduced, such legislation is to be referred to the Senate Committee on Finance and to the House Committees on Energy and Commerce and Ways and Means. These committees may mark up the measure, and must report it to their respective chambers not later than April 1 or be discharged of its further consideration. The expedited procedure waives the provisions of Senate Rule XV, which would ordinarily bar the Finance Committee from reporting a committee amendment containing significant matter not in its jurisdiction so long as the amendment in question "is relevant" to a proposal in the Advisory Board bill.

The provision also restricts the House or Senate from considering any amendment (including committee amendment), bill, or conference report which would repeal or change the Board's recommendations unless those changes meet the same fiscal and policy criteria (described above) that the Board was required to meet in developing its recommendations. PPACA provides for this restriction to apply not only to House and Senate consideration of the Board legislation submitted by the President, but to all other legislation Congress considers as well. This restriction may be waived solely by a vote of three-fifths of the Members.

No expedited procedures are established for initial House floor consideration of the Board's legislation. In the Senate, a motion to proceed to consider the legislation is privileged and not debatable. Amendments offered to the legislation on the Senate floor must be germane and may not reduce the savings in Medicare per capita growth below established targets. Debate in the Senate on each amendment to the bill is limited and overall Senate consideration of the legislation may not exceed 30 hours, after which a final vote will be taken on it. In the event that there is a need to resolve bicameral differences on the legislation, debate on any conference report or amendment exchange is limited to no more than 10 hours, after which a final vote will occur. Should the measure be vetoed, Senate debate on a veto message is limited to one hour.

Fast Track Consideration of Legislation to Discontinue Payment Advisory Board. The provision establishes an additional set of fast track parliamentary procedures governing House and Senate consideration of a joint resolution to discontinue the Independent Payment Advisory Board and the "automatic" process of implementation described above. These procedures ensure that the House and Senate may act promptly on such a measure by limiting debate and amendment at the committee and floor level. The procedures also establish a supermajority requirement of three-fifths of Members duly chosen and sworn for passage of such a joint resolution in each chamber.[56]

Implementation by the Secretary. The Secretary is required to implement the Board's recommendations by August 15 of the year in which the proposal was submitted. Any recommendation that would change a provider's payment rate will apply on the first day of the first fiscal year, calendar year, or rate year (which varies depending on provider type) after August 15th.

Beginning in 2019, the Secretary will be prohibited from implementing the Board's recommendations if two conditions are met: (1) the Board was required to submit a proposal to Congress in the preceding year, and (2) the OACT determined that the rate of growth in per capita NHE exceeded the rate of growth in per capita Medicare spending. These restrictions are not to affect requirements pertaining to the Board's submission of proposals to Congress or the rules related to congressional consideration of these proposals.

Additional Review Procedures. The Board must submit a draft copy of each proposal it develops to the Medicare Payment Advisory Commission (MedPAC) and to the Secretary for review.

Advisory Functions. Beginning in 2014, for any year the Board is not required to submit a proposal to the President and Congress, the Board will be required to submit to Congress advisory reports on matters related to the Medicare program. Prior to 2020, these reports may include recommendations to improve payment systems for those providers and suppliers exempted from the Board's recommendations.

Beginning in 2015, the provision also requires that the Board submit to Congress and the President advisory recommendations to slow the rate of growth in NHE. These recommendations could not target expenditures in federal health care programs. The Board will be required to coordinate these recommendations, which must be made available to the public, with those contained in other Board proposals and advisory reports. Recommendations, which are required at a minimum once every two years, could be implemented either administratively by the Secretary or legislatively by Congress. These advisory reports will not be subject to the rules for congressional consideration.

Funding. The provision appropriates $15 million to the Board to carry out its functions beginning in year 2012. This amount will increase by the rate of inflation for each year thereafter. Sixty percent of the appropriation will come from the Part A Medicare Trust Fund and 40% from the Part B Trust Fund.

Oversight Mechanisms. The provision establishes a consumer advisory council to advise the Board on the impact of payment policies on consumers. The Council is to be composed of 10 consumer representatives appointed by the Comptroller General of the United States, each from among the 10 regions established by the Secretary. The provision also requires the GAO to conduct a study on changes in payment policies, methodologies, rates, and coverage policies under Medicare resulting from the Board's proposal. Specifically, the study is to provide an assessment of the effect of the Board's proposal on Medicare beneficiary's access to providers, affordability of premiums and cost-sharing, the potential impact of changes on other government or private sector purchasers of care, and the quality of care provided. The report is due by July 1, 2015. The GAO is to conduct additional studies as appropriate. *The CBO score is $0.0 billion for FY2010-FY2014 and -$15.5 billion for FY2015-FY2019.*[57]

Subtitle G—Protecting and Improving Guaranteed Medicare Benefits

Sec. 3601. Protecting and Improving Guaranteed Medicare Benefits. This section requires that that no provisions in PPACA may result in a reduction in Medicare benefits currently guaranteed under Title XVIII. This section also requires that Medicare savings achieved under the PPACA are to be used to extend the solvency of the Medicare trust funds, reduce Medicare premiums and other cost-sharing for beneficiaries, improve or expand guaranteed Medicare benefits, and protect access to Medicare providers. *This provision was not scored by CBO.*

Sec. 3602. No Cuts in Guaranteed Benefits. Under prior law, MA plans were required to provide all Medicare covered benefit except hospice. This provision requires that nothing in the PPACA may result in the reduction or elimination of any benefits guaranteed by law to participants in Medicare Advantage plans. *This provision was not scored by CBO.*

Title IV—Prevention of Chronic Disease and Improving Public Health

Subtitle B—Increasing Access to Clinical Prevention Services.[58]

Sec. 4103 as modified by 10402(b). Medicare Coverage of Annual Wellness Visit Providing a Personalized Prevention Plan.[59] Medicare covers a one-time initial preventive physical examination (IPPE), for purposes of health promotion and disease detection, which includes education, counseling, and referrals with respect to screening and other preventive services. The IPPE is reimbursable only if provided within one year of Medicare Part B enrollment. Medicare does not otherwise cover periodic routine health examinations (i.e., those provided in the absence of symptoms).

The U.S. Preventive Services Task Force (USPSTF), administered by the HHS Agency for Healthcare Research and Quality (AHRQ), is an independent panel of private-sector experts in primary care and prevention that conducts assessments of scientific evidence of the effectiveness of a broad range of clinical preventive services, including screening, counseling, and preventive medications.[60] It provides evidence-based recommendations for the use of preventive services, which may vary depending on age, gender, and risk factors for disease, among other considerations. Services are given a grade of A, B, C, D or an I Statement. Services graded A or B are recommended. For services graded C, the USPSTF makes no recommendation for or against their routine use. For services graded D, the USPSTF recommends against routinely providing the service to asymptomatic patients, based on evidence that the service is not beneficial, and may be harmful. "I" Statements are provided when evidence is insufficient to support a recommendation.

This provision amends SSA§1861 to require that Medicare Part B cover, without cost-sharing, "personalized prevention plan services," including a comprehensive health risk assessment beginning on January 1, 2011. The personalized plan can include several specified elements, including medical and family history, identification of health risk factors, and a plan for preventive screenings. All enrolled beneficiaries will be eligible for personalized prevention plan services once every year without any cost-sharing. During the first year of Part B enrollment, beneficiaries can receive only the IPPE. Beneficiaries will be eligible to receive personalized prevention plan services each year thereafter provided that the beneficiary has not received either an IPPE or personalized prevention plan services within the preceding 12 months. The Secretary is required to develop appropriate guidance and conduct outreach and related activities with respect to personalized prevention plan services and health risk assessments. These services are included in the list of Medicare covered preventive services under Sec. 4104 of PPACA. *The CBO score is $1.4 billion for FY2010-FY2014 and $3.6 billion for FY2010-FY2019.*

Sec. 4104. Removal of Barriers to Preventive Services in Medicare. Section 1833(a) of the SSA establishes coinsurance for the beneficiary, generally requiring Medicare to cover 80% of the costs of covered services under Part B, with specified exceptions. Section 1833(b) establishes an annual deductible for which the beneficiary is responsible. These sections have been amended over the years to waive coinsurance and/or the deductible for many, but not all, covered preventive services.

The provision amends SSA Sec. 1861 to define preventive services covered by Medicare to mean a specified list of currently covered services, including colorectal cancer screening services even if diagnostic or treatment services were furnished in connection with the screening. The list also includes the IPPE, as well as the personalized prevention plan services that are covered pursuant to Sec. 4103 of PPACA. Coverage will continue to be subject to all criteria that apply to each preventive service covered under prior law. The provision also amends SSA Sec. 1833 to waive beneficiary coinsurance requirements for most preventive services, requiring Medicare to cover 100% of the costs. Services for which no coinsurance will be required are the IPPE, personalized prevention plan services, any additional preventive service covered under the Secretary's administrative authority, and any currently covered preventive service (including medical nutrition therapy, and excluding electrocardiograms) if it is recommended with a grade of A or B by the USPSTF. The provision generally waives the application of the deductible for the same types of preventive services noted above for which coinsurance would be waived. It does not, however, waive the application of the deductible for any additional preventive service covered under the Secretary's administrative authority. *The CBO score is $0.3 billion for FY2010-FY2014 and $0.8 billion for FY2010-FY2019.*

Sec. 4105. Evidence-Based Coverage of Medicare Preventive Services. The provision authorizes the Secretary to modify the coverage of any currently covered preventive service (including services included in the IPPE, but not the IPPE itself), to the extent that the modification is consistent with USPSTF recommendations. The provision also allows the Secretary to withhold payment for any currently covered preventive service graded D (i.e., not recommended) by the USPSTF. The enhanced authority and the prohibition do not apply to services furnished for the purposes of diagnosis or treatment (rather than as preventive services furnished to asymptomatic patients). *The CBO score is -$0.3 billion for FY2010-FY2014 and -$0.7 billion for FY2010-FY2019.*

Subtitle C—Creating Healthier Communities

Sec. 4202. Medicare Demonstration: Promotion of Healthy Lifestyles. Subsection (b) of this provision requires the Secretary to conduct an evaluation of community-based prevention and wellness programs, and based on findings, develop a plan for promoting healthy lifestyles and chronic disease self-management for Medicare beneficiaries. The evaluation is to include an evidence review of literature, best practices, and resources, and an evaluation of existing community prevention and wellness programs sponsored by the Administration on Aging. To fund the evaluation, the Secretary is required to transfer to CMS $50 million in total from the Part A and Part B Trust Funds, in whatever proportion the Secretary determines. Activities under this evaluation will not be subject to review under the Paperwork Reduction Act of 1995, which subjects collections of information from the public to clearance by OMB. *The CBO score is $0.1 billion for FY2010-FY2014 and $0.1 billion for FY2010-FY2019.*

Sec. 4204. Immunizations. Among other requirements, this section requires GAO to conduct a study and report to Congress on the impact of the coverage of vaccines under Medicare Part D on access to those vaccines by beneficiaries who are 65 years of age or older. The section appropriates $1 million for FY2010 for this study. *The CBO score is $0.0 for FY2010-FY2014 and $0.0 for FY2010-FY2019.*

Title V—Health Care Workforce

Subtitle F—Strengthening Primary Care and Other Workforce Improvements61

Sec. 5501. Expanding Access to Primary Care Services and General Surgery Services. Medicare uses a fee schedule to reimburse physicians for the services they provide. In certain circumstances, physicians receive an additional payment to encourage targeted activities. These bonuses, typically a percentage increase above the Medicare fee schedule amounts, can be awarded for a number of activities including demonstrating quality achievements, participating in electronic prescribing, or practicing in underserved areas. For instance, Section 1833(m) of the Social Security Act provides bonus payments for physicians who furnish medical care services in geographic areas that are designated by the Health Resources and Services Administration (HRSA) as primary medical care health professional shortage areas (HPSAs) under Section 332 (a)(1)(A) of the Public Health Service (PHS) Act. The bonus payment equals 10% of what would otherwise be paid under the fee schedule.

The provision establishes a new 10% bonus on select evaluation & management (E&M) and general surgery codes under the Medicare fee schedule for five years, beginning January 1, 2011. The primary care service codes to which this bonus applies will be office visits, nursing facility visits, and home visits. The bonus will be available to primary care practitioners who (1) are physicians who have a specialty designation of family medicine, internal medicine, geriatric medicine, or pediatric medicine, or are nurse practitioners, clinical nurse specialists, or physician assistants, and (2) furnish 60% of their services in the select codes.

Practitioners providing major surgical procedures in health professional shortage areas will also be eligible for a bonus under this provision. Over the same five year period beginning January 1, 2011, general surgeons providing care in a HPSA will be eligible for a 10% bonus on major surgical procedure codes, defined as surgical procedures for which a 10-day or 90-day global period is used for payment under the Medicare fee schedule.

The review and adjustment of RVUs (under Section 1848(c)(2)(B)) will be adjusted for these incentives; only half (50%) of the cost of the bonuses are to be taken into consideration in the budget neutrality calculation in 2011 and in subsequent years, with an across-the-board reduction to all codes (through a modification of the conversion factor) accounting for the adjustment, except for physicians who primarily provide services in health professionals shortage areas. *The CBO score is $2.5 billion for FY2010-FY2014 and is $3.5 billion for FY2010-FY2019.*

Sec. 10501(i). Development and Implementation of Prospective Payment System (PPS) for FQHCs. A federally qualified health center (FQHC) is a type of provider defined by the Medicare and Medicaid statutes. FQHCs include all organizations receiving grants under section 330 of the Public Health Service Act (PHSA), clinics that have been certified as meeting such requirements (called FQHC Look-Alikes) or outpatient facilities that are operated by tribal organization or urban Indian organizations. FQHC services are defined by Medicare statute as rural health clinic services (such as physician services, those provided by physician assistants, nurse practitioners, nurse midwives, visiting nurses, clinical psychologist or social workers and related services and supplies), diabetes outpatient self-management training services, medical nutrition therapy services and preventive primary health services required under section 330 of the Public Health Service Act (PHSA).[62]

FQHCs receive cost-based reimbursement from Medicare, subject to a per-visit payment limit and certain productivity standards. Medicare pays FQHCs on an interim basis for covered services furnished to beneficiaries using an all-inclusive rate for each visit (except for certain vaccines which are paid on a cost basis). Generally, the FQHC's final payment rate is calculated by dividing the FQHC's total allowable cost for such services by the total visits which is subject to the maximum per-visit payment limit. The payment limits are increased each year by the Medicare Economic Index (MEI) and are different for urban and rural

FQHCs. The upper payment limit per visit for urban FQHCs is $119.29 starting January 1, 2009, through December 31, 2009, and per visit limit for rural FQHCs is $102.58 effective January 1, 2009.

This provision repealed Sec. 5502 established earlier in the legislation. Under Sec. 10501(i), effective for services starting on January 1, 2011, the statutory definition of FQHC services will include the Medicare definition of preventive services at 1861(ddd)(3) that were established in Section 2002 of PPACA. These services include screening and preventive services (other than electrocardiograms), an initial preventive physical examination, and personalized prevention plan services. The cross reference to preventive services in the PHSA will be retained.

The Secretary is to develop a prospective payment system (PPS) for FQHC services as established by a new Section 1834(o) of the SSA. The PPS will establish payment rates for specific codes that take into account the type, intensity and duration of services and can include appropriate geographic adjusters. FQHCs will be required to submit necessary data no later than January 1, 2011. The new payment system will be established for cost reporting periods beginning on or after October 1, 2014. Initial FQHC payments under the new PPS are to equal 100% of reasonable costs (determined without application of a per visit payment limit or productivity screen) that would have been reimbursed if the PPS system had not been implemented. In subsequent years, payments rates will be increased by the MEI (in the first year) or by a MB promulgated by regulations if available. FQHC payment codes may be implemented by program instruction. Program payments for FQHC services will be made at 80% of the lesser of actual charge or the PPS amount. FQHCs that contract with MA plans will receive what they would otherwise receive under the new PPS. Medicare's payments for FQHCs services will no longer be subject to reasonableness tests. *CBO did not provide a separate score for this subsection of the provision.*

Title VI—Transparency and Program Integrity

Subtitle A—Physician Ownership and Other Transparency

Sec. 6001 as modified by Sec. 10601 of PPACA, and by Sec. 1106 of the Reconciliation Act. Limitation on Medicare Exception to the Prohibition on Certain Physician Referrals for Hospitals. Physicians are generally prohibited from referring Medicare patients for certain services to facilities in which they (or their immediate family members) have financial interests. However, among other exceptions, physicians are not prohibited from referring patients to whole hospitals in which they have ownership or investment interests. Providers that furnish substantially all of their designated health services to individuals residing in rural areas are exempt as well. Under this provision, beginning no later than 18 months after the date of enactment, only physician-owned hospitals meeting certain requirements will be exempt from the prohibition on self-referral. Hospitals that have physician ownership and a provider agreement in operation on December 31, 2010, and that meet other specified requirements will be exempt from this self-referral ban. These requirements include a limitation on the expansion of the facilities' service capacity and address conflicts of interest, bona fide investments, and patient safety issues. In addition, the hospital could not have converted from an ambulatory surgical center to a hospital after the date of enactment.

Exempt hospitals meeting those requirements will not be permitted to increase the number of operating rooms, procedure rooms or beds for which the hospital is licensed as the date of enactment. A process is to be established to allow certain hospitals to expand by February 1, 2011, as established by regulations promulgated by January 1, 2011. Hospitals can apply for such an expansion once every two years. The increase will be limited to facilities on the main campus of the hospital. There will be no administrative or judicial review of this process. The Secretary is required to establish policies and procedures to ensure compliance with these requirements, beginning on their effective date, including unannounced site reviews of hospitals. These audits are to begin no later than May 1, 2012. *The CBO score is -$0.1 billion for FY2010-FY2014 and -$0.5 billion for FY2010-FY2019.*

Sec. 6002. Transparency Reports and Reporting of Physician Ownership or Investment Interests. This provision adds a new section 1128G to the Social Security Act to require covered drug, device, biological, or medical supply manufacturers that make a payment or another transfer of value to a physician (other than employees of a manufacturer) or a teaching hospital to report annually, in electronic form, specified information on such transactions to the Secretary of HHS. Certain information is to be excluded from these reporting requirements, including payments or transfers of $10 or less, unless the aggregate annual payments or transfers to a recipient exceeds $100 (which, after 2012, would be indexed for inflation), samples intended for patient use, patient educational materials, and loans of a covered device for a short-term time period. The provision also requires manufacturers, or group purchasing organizations to report annually to the Secretary, in electronic form, certain information regarding an ownership or investment interest held by a physician (or an immediate family member) in the manufacturer or group purchasing organization during the preceding year. Certain penalties will apply for failure to submit these reports to the Secretary. The Secretary is also required to establish procedures to ensure public availability of the information to be submitted under this section. *The CBO score is $0.0 billion for FY2010-FY2014 and $0.0 billion for FY2010-FY2019.*

Sec. 6003. Disclosure Requirements for In-Office Ancillary Services Exception to the Prohibition on Physician Self-Referral for Certain Imaging Services. This section amends section 1877 of the Social Security Act, which prohibits physician referrals, for certain services that may be paid for by Medicare, to entities with which the physician has a financial relationship. Specifically, section 6003 amends one of the exceptions to this prohibition, the in-office ancillary services exception. The provision adds a requirement that with respect to magnetic resonance imaging, computed tomography, positron emission tomography, and any other designated health services as determined by the Secretary, the referring physician must inform the individual in writing at the time of the referral that the individual may obtain the services from a person other than the referring physician, a physician who is a member of the same group practice as the referring physician, or an individual who is directly supervised by the physician or by another physician in the group practice. The individual must be provided with a written list of suppliers who furnish these services in the area in which the individual resides. *The CBO score is $0.0 billion for FY2010-FY2014 and $0.0 billion for FY2010-FY2019.*

Sec. 6004. Prescription Drug Sample Transparency. The provision adds a new section 1128H of the Social Security Act to require drug manufacturers and authorized distributors of an applicable drug to submit annually to the Secretary of Department of Health and Human Services the identity and quantity of drug samples requested and distributed under section 503 of the Prescription Drug Marketing Act of 1987 (PDMA, P.L. 100-293). This submission must be aggregated by the name, address, professional designation, and signature or the practitioner making the request for the sample (or an individual acting on the practitioner's behalf), as well as any other category of information that the Secretary determines is appropriate. An applicable drug is defined to include drugs that are available by prescription and for which payment is available under Medicare or a Medicaid state plan (or a waiver of such plan). *The CBO score is $0.0 billion for FY2010-FY2014 and $0.0 billion for FY2010-FY2019.*

Sec. 6005. Pharmacy Benefit Managers Transparency Requirements. Pharmacy benefit managers (PBMs) are companies that administer drug benefit programs for employers and health insurance carriers. Drug manufacturers may provide "rebates" to PBMs for a particular drug in exchange for the placement of the drug on the PBM's formulary (it's list of approved drugs). This provision requires PBMs that manage prescription drug coverage under a contract with a Part D drug plan or a qualified health plan offered through an exchange (established by a state under Section 1311 of PPACA) to share certain financial information with the Secretary of HHS, the plans the PBMs contract with through Medicare Part D, or the exchanges in a manner, form, and timeframe specified by the Secretary. Specifically, PBMs are required to disclose information on: (1) the percentage of all prescriptions that are provided through retail pharmacies compared to mail order pharmacies, and the generic dispensing rates for each type of pharmacy (for example, independent, chain, supermarket or mass merchandiser pharmacy) that is paid by the PBM under contract; (2) the aggregate amount and types of rebates, discounts or price concessions that the PBM negotiates on behalf of the plan and the aggregate amount of these that are passed through to the plan sponsor, and the total number of prescriptions dispensed; and (3) the aggregate amount of the difference between the amount the plan pays the PBM and the amount that the PBM pays the retail and mail order pharmacy, and the total number of prescriptions dispensed. This information is considered confidential and is to be protected by the Secretary. *The CBO score is $0.0 billion for FY2010-FY2014 and $0.0 billion for FY2010-FY2019.*[63]

Subtitle D—Patient-Centered Outcomes Research

Sec. 6301. Patient-Centered Outcomes Research as modified by Sec. 10602. The need for credible information about which clinical strategies work best, under what circumstances and for whom has been widely recognized by clinicians, patients, researchers and policy makers. Commonly referred to as comparative effectiveness research (CER), the Institute of Medicine (IOM) defines this type of research as the "the generation and synthesis of evidence that compares the benefits and harms of alternative methods to prevent, diagnose, treat, monitor a clinical condition and improve delivery of care" with the aim of tailoring decisions to the needs of individual patients. CBO has referred to CER as "a comparison of the impact of different options that are available for treating a given medical condition for a particular set of patients." MedPAC has referred to "comparative-effectiveness" as "analysis [that] compares the clinical effectiveness of a service (drugs, devices, diagnostic and surgical procedures, diagnostic tests, and medical services) with its alternatives." The phrase "patient-centered outcomes research" has also been used as an alternate term.

Most recently, comparative effectiveness research has been addressed in current law by the Medicare Prescription Drug, Improvement, and Modernization Act of 2003 (MMA, P.L. 108-173) and the American Recovery and Reinvestment Act of 2009 (ARRA, P.L. 111-5). Section 1013 of the MMA authorizes the Agency for Healthcare Research and Quality (AHRQ) to conduct and support research on outcomes, comparative clinical effectiveness, and appropriateness of pharmaceuticals, devices, and health care services. The section also prohibits the Center for Medicare and Medicaid Services (CMS) from using the data to withhold coverage of a prescription drug. The ARRA provided $1.1 billion in funds to support the development and dissemination of CER. ARRA also asked the Institute of Medicine to recommend national priorities for the research to be addressed by ARRA funds.

This section of the PPACA modifies Title XI of the Social Security Act to add a Part D, Comparative Clinical Effectiveness Research after sections on General Provisions, Peer Review, and Administrative Simplification. The provision authorizes the establishment of a private, nonprofit, tax-exempt corporation, which is to be neither an agency nor establishment of the United States government called the "Patient-Centered Outcomes Research Institute." This institute is to enhance the capacity to conduct comparative clinical effectiveness research (CCER). The purpose of the Institute would be to "assist patients, clinicians, purchasers, and policy makers in making informed health decisions by advancing the quality and relevance of evidence concerning the manner in which diseases, disorders, and other health conditions can effectively and appropriately be prevented, diagnosed, treated, monitored, and managed through research and evidence synthesis that considers variations in patient sub-populations, and the dissemination of research findings with respect to the relative health outcomes, clinical effectiveness, and appropriateness of the medical treatments, services, and items."

The duties of the Institute are to (1) identify research priorities and establish a research agenda, (2) carry out the research project agenda, (3) collect relevant data from CMS and other sources, (4) appoint expert advisory panels, (5) support patient and consumer representatives, (6) establish a methodology committee, (7) provide for a peer-review process for primary research, (8) release research findings, (9) adopt the national priorities, the research project agenda, the methodological standards developed and updated by the methodology committee, and any peer-review process provided under point (7), and (10) submit an annual report to Congress and the President. The Institute is to give preference to the Agency for Healthcare Research and Quality and the National Institutes of Health in the awarding of contracts to conduct the research, if the organizations are so authorized in their governing statutes.

The provision establishes a Board of Governors for the Institute, which would be responsible for carrying out the duties of the Institute. The Institute's Board is to consist of the Directors of AHRQ and the NIH (or their designee) as well as 17 members appointed by the Comptroller General of the United States representing patients and health care consumers, physicians and providers, private payers, pharmaceutical, device, and diagnostic manufacturers or developers, representatives of quality improvement or independent health service researchers, and representatives of the federal government or the states.

The provision includes a number of limitations on the use of CCER. A rule of construction specifies that the Institute is not to be permitted to mandate coverage, reimbursement or other policies for any public or private payer nor to prevent the Secretary from covering the routine costs of clinical care received by Medicare, Medicaid, or CHIP beneficiaries in the case where the individual is participating in a clinical trial where the costs would be covered by the program. In addition, the Secretary could only use evidence and findings from CCER to make a Medicare coverage determination if the process is iterative and transparent and includes public comment and considers the effect on subpopulations.

CCER is not to be construed as (1) superseding or modifying the coverage of items or services under Medicare that the Secretary determines are reasonable and necessary, nor (2) authorizing the Secretary to deny coverage of items or services under Medicare solely on the basis of comparative clinical effectiveness research. The Secretary is prohibited from using CCER evidence and findings in determining Medicare coverage, reimbursement, or incentive programs in a manner that treats extending the life of an elderly, disabled, or terminally ill individual as of lower value than extending the life of an individual who is younger, non-disabled, or not terminally ill, nor in a manner that would preclude or have the intent to discourage individuals from choosing health care treatments based on how the individual values the tradeoff between extending the length of life and the risk of disability. The Institute will also not be allowed to develop or employ a dollars-per-quality adjusted life year or similar measure that discounts value of life because of disability as a threshold to establish what type of care is cost effective or recommended, nor would the Secretary utilize such an adjusted life year (or such a similar measure) as a threshold to determine coverage, reimbursement, or incentive programs under Medicare.

The provision creates a new trust fund, the Patient-Centered Outcomes Research Trust Fund (the PCORTF) in the U.S. Treasury to fund the Institute and its activities. Monies will be directed to this fund from the general fund of the Treasury as well as the Medicare Trust Funds and from fees imposed on health insurance and self-insured plans. In years 2010, 2011, and 2012, $10 million, $50 million, and $150 million will be appropriated from Treasury to the fund.

Beginning in 2013, the PCORTF will also be financed from fees on health insurance and self-insured health plans. For FY2013, the Secretary will transfer amounts from the Medicare Federal Hospital Insurance and the Federal Supplemental Medical Trust Funds to the PCORTF in proportion to total Medicare expenditures that come from each Fund for a given year. In FY2013, the amount is to be equivalent to $1 multiplied by the average number of individuals entitled to benefits under Part A or enrolled under Part B of Medicare during the year. (In FY2014 through FY2019, the amounts are to be equivalent to $2, adjusted for increases in health care spending FY2014, multiplied by the average number of such individuals for the given year.)

For fiscal years 2014 through 2019, the provision requires a transfer of $150 million from the Treasury as well as the net revenues from a fee of $1 in FY2013 and $2 (adjusted for health care spending increases) in FY2014 through FY2019, on each health insurance policy in the United States multiplied by the number of lives covered under that policy. Insurance policies that primarily provide non-health benefits will be exempt. This fee will sunset after FY2019 (plan years ending after September 30, 2019). *The CBO score is $0.1 billion for FY2010-FY2014 and -$0.3 billion for FY2010-FY2019.*

Subtitle E—Medicare, Medicaid, and CHIP Program Integrity Provisions

Sec. 6401 as modified by Sec. 10603 of PPACA, and Sec. 1304 of the Reconciliation Act. Provider Screening and Other Enrollment Requirements Under Medicare, Medicaid, and CHIP. CMS has implemented regulations requiring providers and suppliers to complete an application to enroll in the Medicare program and receive billing privileges. As part of the enrollment process, providers and suppliers are required to submit information necessary to verify identity and state licensure. CMS reserves the right to perform on-site inspections of a provider or supplier to verify compliance with standards. If enrollment requirements are not met, CMS may revoke Medicare billing privileges. Providers and suppliers must resubmit and recertify the accuracy of their enrollment information every five years. This provision requires the Secretary to establish procedures for enrolling providers and suppliers enrolling in the Medicare, Medicaid, and CHIP programs. The enrollment process is required to include provider screening, enhanced oversight measures, disclosure requirements, moratoriums on enrollment, and requirements for developing compliance programs.

Provider Screening. The Secretary, in consultation with the OIG, has six months to develop the procedures related to provider screening. The Secretary is to determine the level of screening according to risk and with respect to a category of providers and suppliers. At a minimum, all providers and suppliers will be subject to licensure checks, including checks across states. The Secretary has the authority to impose additional screening measures such as criminal background checks, fingerprinting, unannounced site visits, database checks, and other screening measures as appropriate. To cover the costs of screening, institutional providers will be subject to fees. Fees will start at $500 in 2010 and increase by the rate of inflation annually thereafter. The provision requires the Secretary to use the fees collected to fund program integrity efforts. The Secretary has the authority to exempt providers from fees in case of hardship. The revised screening measures will apply to providers and suppliers who have not yet enrolled in Medicare, Medicaid, and CHIP in one year, to current providers and suppliers in two years, and to providers and suppliers re-enrolling in one or more of these programs in 6 months. No provider or supplier will be allowed to participate in Medicare, Medicaid, or CHIP if they have not been screened within three years.

Enhanced Oversight. The Secretary is required to establish procedures for imposing periods of enhanced oversight, such as prepayment review and payment caps, on new providers and suppliers. The period cannot be less than 30 days or last more than one year. Beginning January 1, 2011, in instance when there is a significant risk of fraud, the Secretary will be required to impose a 90-day period of enhanced oversight on DME suppliers initially enrolling in the program. The Secretary will also have the authority to impose temporary moratoriums on enrolling new providers and suppliers if the Secretary determines that these moratoriums are necessary to combat fraud.

Disclosure Requirements. The provision imposes new disclosure requirements on providers and suppliers enrolling or re-enrolling in Medicare, Medicaid, or CHIP. Applicants will be required to disclose current or previous affiliations with any provider or supplier that has uncollected debt, has had their payments suspended, has been excluded from participating in Medicare, Medicaid, or CHIP, or has had their billing privileges revoked. The Secretary is authorized to adjust payments or deny enrollment in these programs if these affiliations pose an undue risk to the program.

Compliance Programs. The provision requires Medicare, Medicaid, and CHIP providers and suppliers, within a particular industry or category, to establish a compliance program. The requirements for the compliance program are to be developed by the Secretary and the OIG. The Secretary is required to consider the extent to which compliance programs have been adopted by providers when creating a timeline for implementation. *The CBO score is $0.0 for FY2010-FY2014 and -$0.1 billion for FY2010-FY2019.*

Sec. 6402 as modified by Sec. 1303 of the Reconciliation Act. Enhanced Medicare and Medicaid Program Integrity Provisions.

Data Matching. Currently, claims and payment data for Medicare and Medicaid are housed in multiple databases. CMS is in the process of consolidating information stored in these databases into an Integrated Data Repository (IDR). According to the agency's website, the eventual goal of the IDR is to support an integrated data warehouse containing data related to Medicare & Medicaid claims, beneficiaries, providers, and health plans. The provision requires CMS to include in the IDR claims and payment data from the following programs: Medicare (Parts A, B, C, and D), Medicaid, CHIP, health-related programs administered by the Departments of Veterans Affairs (VA) and Defense (DOD), Social Security, and the Indian Health Service (IHS). The priority is the integration of Medicare and Medicaid claims and payment data. Data for the remaining programs is to be integrated as appropriate. The Secretary is required to enter into data sharing agreements with the federal agencies listed above for the purposes of identifying fraud, waste, and abuse. This provision also grants the OIG and the DOJ explicit access to Medicare, Medicaid, and CHIP payment and claims data (including Medicare Part D data) for the purposes of conducting law enforcement and oversight activities.

Access to Data. Inspectors General have substantial independence and powers to carry out their mandate to combat waste, fraud, and abuse, including relatively unlimited authority to access all records and information of an agency. This provision grants the OIG the authority, under Medicare and Medicaid, to obtain information from any individual (including a beneficiary) or entity (i.e., provider, supplier, contractor, subcontractor, etc.) that directly or indirectly provides medical services payable by a Federal health care program. Types of information include any supporting documentation necessary to validate a claim for payment such as medical records for individuals prescribed Medicare Part B or Part D drugs. PPACA includes a separate clause mandating that the HHS OIG, the DOJ, and the GAO have access to Medicare Part D data for the purposes of carrying out health oversight activities.

Beneficiary Participation in Health Care Fraud Scheme. The provision requires the Secretary to impose penalties against beneficiaries entitled to or enrolled in Medicare, Medicaid, or CHIP who knowingly participate in a health care fraud offense.

Overpayments. In accordance with CMS instructions, overpayments must be repaid to CMS within 30 days of receiving a demand letter. If the debt is not paid in full after 30 days, interest is assessed and CMS reserves the right to collect the overpayment by offset. Under this provision, individuals will be required to report and return an overpayment within 60 days. Overpayments reported after this date will be considered an obligation as defined in Title 31 of the USC.

National Provider Identifier. Health care providers often have many different provider numbers, one for billing each private insurance plan or public health care program. The administrative simplification provisions of HIPAA required the adoption and use of a standard unique identifier for health care providers or National Provider Identifier (NPI). All health care providers who are considered covered entities under HIPAA were required to obtain and submit claims using an NPI as of May 2007. This provision requires the Secretary to issue a regulation by January 1, 2011, mandating that all Medicare and Medicaid providers include their NPI on all claims and enrollment applications.

Permissive Exclusions. HHS OIG has the authority to exclude health care providers from participation in federal health care programs. Exclusions are mandatory under certain circumstances, and permissive in others (i.e., HHS OIG has discretion in whether to exclude an entity or individual). This provision subjects any individual or entity that makes a false statement or misrepresentation on an application to enroll or participate in a federal health care program to the OIG's permissive exclusion authority. The provision explicitly applies to MA plans, Medicare prescription drug plans (PDPs), and Medicaid managed care plans as well as their participating providers and suppliers.

Civil Monetary Penalties (CMPs). Section 1128A (a) of the SSA authorizes the imposition of CMPs on a person, organization, agency, or other entity that engages in various types of improper conduct with respect to federal health care programs. This section generally provides for CMPs of up to $10,000 for each false claim submitted, $15,000 or $50,000 under other circumstances, and an assessment of up to three times the amount claimed. This provision adds additional actions that are subject to CMPs. Specifically, individuals who have been excluded from a Federal health care program who order or prescribe an item or service; individuals who make false statements on enrollment applications, bids, or contracts to participate in a federal health care program; or persons who know of an overpayment and do not return the overpayment may be subject to a CMPs of $50,000.

Kickbacks and Revising the Intent Requirement. Under the federal anti-kickback statute, SSA Section 1128B(b), it is a felony for a person to knowingly and willfully offer, pay, solicit, or receive anything of value (i.e., "remuneration"), in return for a referral or to induce generation of business reimbursable under a federal health care program. Violations of section 1128B carry penalties of up to $25,000, imprisonment of five years, or both.

The federal False Claims Act (FCA)[64] is considered by many to be an important tool for combating fraud against the U.S. government. In general, the FCA imposes civil liability on persons who knowingly submit a false or fraudulent claim or engage in various improper activities involving federal government money or property. Penalties under the FCA include treble damages, plus an additional penalty of $5,500 to $11,000 for each false claim filed.

Section 6402(f)(1) of PPACA amends section 1128B to provide that a claim for items or services resulting from a violation of section 1128B will also constitute a false or fraudulent claim that may be subject to penalties under the FCA. Further, section 6402(f)(2) of PPACA addresses the intent requirements of section 1128B. This section amends section 1128B to specify that with respect to violations of the section, a person does not have to have actual knowledge of section 1128B, or specific intent to commit a violation of it.

Treatment of Certain Charitable and Other Innocuous Programs. Under Section 1128A of the SSA, the HHS OIG is authorized to impose CMPs and assessments on a person, including an organization, agency, or other entity, who engages in various types of improper conduct with respect to federal health care programs.[65] One type of prohibited conduct, described in section 1128A(a)(5), occurs when a person offers or transfers remuneration to a Medicare or Medicaid beneficiary when such person knows or should know the remuneration is likely to influence the beneficiary's ordering or receiving items or services (payable, at least in part, by Medicare or Medicaid) from a particular provider, practitioner, or supplier. Further, individuals who commit violations of the federal anti-kickback statute,[66] Section 1128B(b), may be subject to CMPs under section 1128A for damages amounting to not more than three times the total amount of remuneration offered, paid, solicited, or received, without regard to whether a portion of such remuneration was offered, paid, solicited, or received for a lawful purpose.

Section 6402(d)(2)(B) of PPACA amends the definition of "remuneration" in section 1128A(i)(6) of the SSA to exclude remuneration that promotes access to care and poses a low risk of harm to patients and federal health care programs; the offer or transfer of items or services for free or less than fair market value by a person, subject to certain additional requirements; and, effective on a date specified by the Secretary (but no earlier than January 1, 2011), a waiver of the copayment amount (under prescription drug plan offered by a PDP sponsor or an MA-PD plan offered by an MA organization) for the first fill of a covered part D drug that is a generic drug for individuals enrolled in a the prescription drug plan or a MA-PD drug plan.

Testimonial Subpoena Authority. The testimonial subpoena authority grants the authority to issue subpoenas and require the attendance and testimony of witnesses and the production of any other evidence that relates to matters under investigation or in question. Under this provision, the Secretary is given the authority to issue subpoenas and require the attendance and testimony of witnesses and the production of any other evidence that relates to matters under investigation or in question by the Secretary. The Secretary also has the ability to delegate this authority to the OIG and the Administrator of CMS for the purposes of a program exclusion investigation.

Surety Bonds. To be eligible to receive a provider number from CMS and bill Medicare, DME suppliers are required to provide the Secretary with a surety bond in the amount of $50,000 or greater. A surety bond issued by a State would satisfy this requirement. The Secretary has the authority to impose these requirements on other Part A and B providers and suppliers, except physicians. Home health agencies are required to provide the Secretary with a surety bond equal to 10% of the aggregate Medicare and Medicaid payments made to the agency for that year or $50,000, whichever is smaller. A surety bond for a home health agency is effective for four years, with limited exceptions. This provision gives the Secretary the authority to require certain providers and suppliers to provide surety bonds commensurate with the volume of billing. The value of the bond, however, cannot be less than $50,000. The Secretary also has the authority to impose this requirement on other providers and suppliers considered to be at risk by the Secretary.

Payment Suspensions. Under CMS regulations, CMS and its contractors have the authority to withhold payment in whole or in part if there is reliable evidence of an overpayment or fraud. CMS regulations stipulate the procedures CMS and its contractors must follow when deciding to suspend payment. This provision provides the Secretary with explicit *statutory* authority to suspend payments to providers and suppliers pending an investigation of fraud, unless the Secretary determines that there is good cause not to suspend payments. The provision also requires the Secretary to consult with the OIG to determine whether there is a credible allegation of fraud and requires the Secretary to implement this provision through rulemaking.

Health Care Fraud and Abuse Control (HCFAC) Account. Activities to fight health care fraud, waste, and abuse are funded by the Health Care Fraud and Abuse Control (HCFAC) account. The HCFAC account funds two programs: (1) the HCFAC program, which finances the investigative and enforcement activities undertaken by HHS, the OIG, the DOJ, and the FBI, and (2) the Medicare Integrity Program (MIP), which finances the program integrity activities undertaken by CMS contractors. HCFAC was established by HIPAA, which sought to increase and stabilize Federal funding for health care anti-fraud activities. HIPAA appropriated funds to the HCFAC account for years 1997 through 2003. In December 2006, Congress passed the Tax Relief and Health Care Act, or TRHCA, which extended the mandatory annual appropriation for the HCFAC program by a CPI adjustment until 2010. TRHCA did not extend the annual appropriation for MIP. This provision appropriates an additional $10 million annually to the HCFAC program for fiscal years 2011 through 2020. Funds are to be appropriated in the same proportion as allocated in FY2010 and are to be available until expended. The provision also permanently applies the CPI adjustment mandated under TRHCA to the HCFAC program and adds a CPI-adjustment to the MIP program beginning in 2011. Sec. 1303 of the Reconciliation Act appropriates additional funding to the HCFAC program for fiscal years 2011 through 2016: (1) $95 million for FY2011; (2) $55 million for FY2012; (3) $30 million for FY2013 and FY2014; and $20 million for FY2015 and FY2016. Funding is to be available without further appropriation until expended.

Medicare and Medicaid Integrity Programs. Under the Medicare Integrity Program (MIP), CMS contracts with private entities to conduct a variety of activities designed to protect Medicare from fraud, waste, and abuse. Activities include auditing providers, identifying and recovering improper payments, educating providers about fraudulent providers, and instituting a Medicare-Medicaid data matching program. This provision requires MIP contractors to provide the Secretary and the OIG with performance statistics, including the number and amount of overpayments recovered, the number of fraud referrals, and the return on investment for such activities as requested by the Secretary or the OIG. The Secretary is also required to conduct evaluations of eligible entities at least every three years and, beginning in FY2011, submit a report to Congress describing the use and effectiveness of MIP funds. The reports will be due 6 months after the end of each fiscal year. *The CBO score is -$1.1 billion for FY2010-FY2014 and -$2.9 billion for FY2010-FY2019.*

Sec. 10330. Modernizing Computer and Data Systems of CMS to Support Improvements in Care Delivery. The provision requires the Secretary to develop a plan along with a budget to modernize the computer and data systems of CMS. In developing the plan, the Secretary is required to consider how such a system could make data available in a timely and reliable manner to providers and suppliers to support their efforts to better manage and coordinate care, and support consistent evaluations of payment and delivery system reforms. The Secretary is required to post the plan on the CMS website within 9 months from the date this legislation is enacted. *The CBO score is $0.0 billion for FY2010-FY2014 and $0.0 billion for FY2010-FY2019.*

Sec. 6403. Elimination of Duplication Between the Healthcare Integrity and Protection Data Bank (HIPDB) and the National Practitioner Data Bank (NPDB). The HIPAA of 1996 required the Secretary to develop and maintain a national health care fraud and abuse data collection program for the reporting of adverse actions taken against health care providers. This database is called the Healthcare Integrity and Protection Data Bank (HIPDB). The statute requires the following types of health care related adverse actions be reported to the HIPDB - civil judgments, federal or state criminal convictions, actions taken by federal or state licensing agencies, and provider exclusions from Medicare and Medicaid. Only final adverse actions are reportable to the HIPDB. Administrative fines, citations, corrective action plans, and other personnel actions are not reportable except under certain circumstances. Settlements, in which a finding of liability has not been established, are also not reportable. Both federal and state government agencies as well as health plans are required to report to the HIPDB. Prior to the HIPDB, Congress established the National Practitioner Data Bank or NPDB with the Health Care Quality Improvement Act of 1986. The NPDB collects data related to the professional competence of physicians, dentists, and other health care practitioners. The types of information included in the NPDB are medical malpractice payments, certain adverse licensure actions, adverse privilege actions, adverse professional society actions, and exclusions from Medicare and Medicaid. Section 1921 of the SSA expanded the scope of reporting requirements for the NPDB to encompass additional adverse licensure actions and actions taken by State licensing and certification agencies, peer review organizations, and private accreditation organizations. States are required to have a system for reporting adverse actions to the NPDB.

This provision requires the Secretary to maintain a national health care fraud and abuse data collection program for the reporting of certain final adverse actions (excluding settlements in which no findings of liability have been made) taken against health care providers and furnish such information to the NPDB. Information collected in the NPDB is to be available to the agencies and authorities listed under section 1921(b). The Secretary has the authority to establish fees for the disclosure of such information. The provision requires States to have a system for reporting information with respect to any final adverse action taken against a health care provider, supplier, or practitioner. The Secretary is also required to implement a transition process, which must be completed within one year, for transferring all information collected in the HIPDB to the NPDB, thereby eliminating the HIPDB. *The CBO score is $0.0 billion for FY2010-FY2014 and $0.0 billion for FY2010-FY2019.*

Sec. 6404. Maximum Period of Submission of Medicare Claims Reduced to Not More Than 12 Months. Prior Medicare statute required that payments only be made if a written request for payment is filed within three calendar years after the year in which the services were provided. The Secretary is authorized to reduce this period to no less than one year if it deems it necessary for the efficient administration of the program. As established by CMS regulations, the time limit on submitting a claim for payment is the close of the calendar year after the year in which the services were furnished. This provision requires that beginning January 2010, the maximum period for submission of Medicare claims be reduced to not more than 12 months. *The CBO score is $0.0 billion for FY2010-FY2014 and $0.0 billion for FY2010-FY2019.*

Sec. 6405 as modified by Sec. 10604. Physicians Who Order Items and Services Required to be Medicare Enrolled Physicians or Eligible Professionals. In order to receive payment from Medicare, physicians are required to certify that specified services (i.e., inpatient psychiatric services, post-hospital extended care services, and home health services) meet certain conditions. In the case of home health services, physicians are required to certify that such services were required because the individual was confined to his home and needs skilled nursing care or physical, speech, or occupational therapy; a plan for furnishing services to the individual has been established; and such services were provided under the care of a physician. In the case of DME, the Secretary is authorized to require, for specified covered items, that payment be made for items and services only if a physician has communicated to the supplier a written order for the item. This provision requires that for written orders and certifications made on or after July 1, 2010, physicians or eligible professionals who order DME or HH services be enrolled in the Medicare program. The Secretary is given the authority to extend these requirements to physicians and eligible professionals that order other categories of Medicare items and services, including covered Part D drugs, if the Secretary determines that it would help reduce fraud, waste, and abuse. *The CBO score is -$0.2 billion for FY2010-FY2014 and -$0.4 billion for FY2010-FY2019.*

Sec. 6406. Requirement for Physicians to Provide Documentation on Referrals to Programs at High Risk of Waste and Abuse. OIG has "permissive" authority to exclude an entity or an individual from a federal health program under numerous circumstances, including failing to supply documentation related to payment for items and services. Under this provision, beginning January 1, 2010, the Secretary has the authority to disenroll, for no more than one year, a Medicare enrolled physician or supplier that fails to maintain and provide access to written orders or requests for payment for DME, certification for home health services, or referrals for other items and services to the Secretary. The provision also extends the OIG's permissive exclusion authority to include individuals or entities that order, refer, or certify the need for health care services that fail to provide adequate documentation to the Secretary to verify payment. *The CBO score is $0.0 billion for FY2010-FY2014 and $0.0 billion for FY2010-FY2019.*

Sec. 6407 as modified by Sec. 10605. Face-to-Face Encounter with Patient Required Before Physicians May Certify Eligibility for Home Health Services or Durable Medical Equipment Under Medicare. Home health services are covered under Medicare Parts A and B. In order to receive payment from Medicare, physicians are required to certify and recertify that specified services (i.e., inpatient psychiatric services, post-hospital extended care services, and home health services) meet certain conditions. In the case of home health services, physicians are required to certify that such services were required because the individual was confined to his home and needs skilled nursing care or physical, speech, or occupational therapy; a plan for furnishing services to the individual has been established; and such services were provided under the care of a physician. In the case of DME, the Secretary is authorized to require, for specified covered items, that payment be made for items and services only if a physician has communicated to the supplier a written order for the item. Under this provision, beginning January 1, 2010, physicians are required to have a face-to-face encounter (including through telehealth) with the individual prior to issuing a certification or re-certification for home health services or DME. Physicians furnishing home health services under Part A are required to document that they had a face-to-face encounter with the patient within a reasonable time frame. Physicians furnishing home health services under Part B are required to document that they had a face-to-face encounter within the six-month period preceding the certification. In the case of DME, physicians are required to document that a physician, physician assistant, nurse practitioner, or clinical nurse specialist have a face-to-face encounter during the six-month period preceding the certification. The Secretary is authorized to apply the face-to-face encounter requirement to other Medicare items and services based upon a finding that doing so would reduce the risk of waste, fraud, and abuse. The provision also specifies that eligible professionals include nurse practitioners or clinical nurse specialists who are collaborating with the physician, a certified nurse midwife, or physician assistant as defined in statute. *The CBO score is -$0.3 billion for FY2010-FY2014 and -$1.0 billion for FY2010-FY2019.*

Sec. 6408. Enhanced Penalties. Section 1128A (a) of the SSA authorizes the imposition of CMPs on a person, organization, agency, or other entity that engages in various types of improper conduct with respect to federal health care programs, and generally provides for CMPs of up to $10,000 for each false claim submitted, $15,000 or $50,000 under other circumstances, and an assessment of up to three times the amount claimed. This provision of PPACA mandates that persons who knowingly make, use, or cause to be made or used any false statement material to a fraudulent claim be subject to a civil monetary penalty of $50,000 for each violation. This provision also adds a new clause to the CMP statute—persons who fail to grant timely access, upon reasonable request (as defined by the Secretary in regulations), to the OIG, for the purpose of audits, investigations, evaluations, or other statutory functions of the OIG, will be subject to CMPs of $15,000 for each day of failure.

Penalties for MA and Part D plans. MA plans enter into contracts with the Secretary to participate in the Medicare program. The Secretary has the authority to impose sanctions and CMPs on MA plans that violate the terms of the contract. Among the types of violations are failing to provide medically necessary care, imposing excess beneficiary premiums, expelling or refusing to re-enroll beneficiaries, and misrepresenting or falsifying information. This provision increases the number of violations subject to sanctions and CMPs by the Secretary. Under the provision, plans that enroll individuals in a MA or Part D plan without their consent (except Part D dual eligibles), transfer an individual from one plan to another for the purpose of earning a commission, fail to comply with marketing requirements, or employ or contract with an individual or entity that violates the terms of the contract will be subject to sanctions imposed by the Secretary. The provision also enhances penalties for plans that misrepresent or falsify information furnished to the Secretary or to an individual by an additional assessment equal to the amount claimed by the plan based on the false information.

These new penalties apply to acts committed on or after January 1, 2010. *The CBO score is $0.0 billion for FY2010-FY2014 and $0.0 billion for FY2010-FY2019.*

Sec. 6409. Medicare Self-Referral Disclosure Protocol. In 1998, the HHS Office of the Inspector General (HHS OIG) issued a Self-Disclosure Protocol (SDP), which includes a process under which a health care provider can voluntarily self-disclose evidence of potential fraud, in an effort, to avoid the costs or disruptions that may be associated with an investigation or litigation. On March 24, 2009, HHS OIG issued an "Open Letter to Health Care Providers" that makes refinements to the SDP. In the Open Letter, HHS OIG announced that it would no longer accept disclosure of a matter that involves only liability under the physician self-referral law in "the absence of a colorable anti-kickback statute violation." Further, for anti-kickback-related submissions accepted into the SDP following the date of the letter, HHS OIG requires a minimum $50,000 settlement amount to resolve the matter. This provision requires that the Secretary, in cooperation with the OIG, establish a self-referral disclosure protocol (SRDP) to enable health care providers and suppliers to disclose actual or potential violations of the physician self-referral law. In addition, the Secretary will be required to post information on CMS' website to inform stakeholders of how to disclose actual or potential SRDP violations. *The CBO score is $0.0 billion for FY2010-FY2014 and $0.0 billion for FY2010-FY2019.*

Sec. 6410. Adjustments to the Medicare Durable Medical Equipment, Prosthetics, Orthotics, and Supplies Competitive Acquisition Program. Medicare generally pays for most durable medical equipment, prosthetics, orthotics and supplies (DMEPOS) on the basis of a fee schedule. MMA required the Secretary to establish a Competitive Acquisition Program for specified medical equipment in specified areas to replace the Medicare fee schedule. The program is to be phased-in, starting in nine of the largest metropolitan statistical areas (MSAs) in 2009 (round 1), expanding to an additional 70 of the largest MSAs in 2011 (round 2) and remaining areas after 2011. PPACA expands the number of areas included in round 2 of the program from 70 to 91 MSAs. The 21 additional MSAs will be the next largest MSAs by population. The Secretary is required to extend the program, or apply competitively bid rates, to remaining areas by 2016. *The CBO score is -$0.3 billion for FY2010-FY2014 and -$1.4 billion for FY2010-FY2019.*

Sec. 6411. Expansion of the Recovery Audit Contractor (RAC) Program. Recovery Audit Contractors, or RACs, are private organizations that contract with CMS to identify and collect improper payments made in Medicare Parts A and B. Congress originally required the Secretary to conduct a three-year demonstration program using RACs in the Medicare Prescription Drug, Improvement, and Modernization Act of 2003 (MMA, P.L. 108-173). In December 2006, Congress passed the Tax Relief and Health Care Act of 2006 (TRHCA, P.L. 109-432), which made the program permanent and mandated the expansion of RACs nationwide by January 1, 2010. Medicare pays RACs differently than it pays other administrative contractors. Historically, Medicare's administrative contractors have been paid a fixed annual budget for a defined scope of work. In contrast, Congress mandated that CMS pay RACs using contingency fees. A contingency fee is a negotiated payment, typically a percentage, for every overpayment recovered. This provision requires that the Secretary enter into contracts with RACs for Medicare Part C and D activities by December 31, 2010. Among the requirements for Part C and D RACs are ensuring that each MA or PDP plan have in place an anti-fraud plan, reviewing the reinsurance payments of Part D plans, and comparing Part D plan's enrollment estimates for high cost beneficiaries. *The CBO score is $0.0 billion for FY2010-FY2014 and $0.0 billion for FY2010-FY2019.*[67]

Sec. 10606. Health Care Fraud Enforcement. This section contains a variety of requirements related to health care fraud enforcement. Among these provisions, the U.S. Sentencing Commission will now be required to review and amend the federal sentencing guidelines and policy statements applicable to persons convicted of federal health care offenses, as specified by the legislation. In addition, PPACA deems existing certain criminal offenses to be "federal health care fraud offenses" under the U.S. Criminal Code.[68] By defining a particular offense as a "federal health care offense," convictions for violations of these listed statutes may be punishable by longer prison terms and/or higher fines, and other enforcement mechanisms may apply.[69] The new federal health care offenses include the federal anti-kickback statute under section 1128B of the Social Security Act (42 U.S.C. § 1320a-7b), section 1349 of the U.S. Criminal Code (attempting or conspiring to commit a criminal offense), section 301 of the Federal Food Drug and Cosmetic Act, and section 501 of ERISA.

This section also amends certain subpoena authority relating to health care. For example, this section amends the Civil Rights of Institutionalized Persons Act (CRIPA, 42 U.S.C. §1997 et seq.), which provides authority for the Department of Justice (DOJ) to initiate or intervene in lawsuits in federal courts in order to protect the rights of institutionalized persons. Under CRIPA, the Attorney General, or a person at his or her direction, could require access by subpoena to any institution that is the subject of an investigation under CRIPA and to additional information relating to any institution that is the subject of an investigation under the Act. The information obtained under a subpoena may not be used for any purpose other than to protect the constitutional and legal rights, privileges, or immunities of persons who reside or will reside in an institution, and the DOJ could not transmit this information for any other purpose. *The CBO score is $0.0 billion for FY2010-FY2014 and $0.0 billion for FY2010-FY2019.*

Sec. 1301 of the Reconciliation Act. Community Mental Health Centers. Under current law, community mental health centers (CMHCs) must meet certain requirements in order to receive payment under Medicare. For example, CMHCs must demonstrate that they can provide the core mental health services described in the Public Health Service Act and that they are licensed in the state in which they are operating. Section 1301 of the Reconciliation Act requires that a CMHC also demonstrate that they provide at least 40% of their services to individuals not eligible for Medicare. Section 1301 also restricts Medicare reimbursement for mental health services delivered in an individual's home or in an inpatient or residential setting.

Sec. 1302 of the Reconciliation Act. Medicare Prepayment Medical Review Limitations. To protect the Medicare program from improper payments and fraudulent billing, Medicare contractors have the authority to review a provider's claims prior to payment. This is referred to as prepayment medical review. Under Medicare statute, contractors can only conduct prepayment review of a provider's claims only under certain circumstances: (1) to develop a claims payment error rate and (2) when there is a likelihood of a sustained or high level of improper billing. Section 1302 of the Reconciliation Act repeals these statutory limitations on prepayment review.

The combined CBO score for1301, 1302, and 1303[70] *is -$0.3 billion for FY2010-FY2014 and -$0.9 billion for FY2010-FY2019.*

Title IX—Revenue Provisions

Subtitle A—Revenue Offset Provisions

Sec. 9015 as modified by Sec. 10906 of PPACA, and Sec. 1402 of the Reconciliation Act. Additional Hospital Insurance Tax on High-Income Taxpayers and Unearned Income Medicare Contribution. Under current law, employees and employers each pay a payroll tax of 1.45% to finance Medicare Part A. PPACA imposes an additional tax of 0.9% on high-income workers with wages over $200,000 for single filers and $250,000 for joint filers effective for taxable years after December 31, 2012. Since employers cannot be expected to know the wages of a spouse, they will be directed to collect these revenues from all workers with wages exceeding $200,000 and then the individuals would have to reconcile any excess withholding on their tax return. The 0.9% tax will also be levied on the self-employed if their incomes exceed the specified thresholds. The self-employed will not be allowed to deduct this additional tax as a business expense.

The Reconciliation Act imposes an additional tax on net investment income, defined as interest, dividends, annuities, royalties, rents and taxable net capital gains. It excludes distributions from a qualified annuity from a pension plan.[71] Households with modified adjusted gross income under these thresholds will not be subject to the investment income tax. Specifically, effective for taxable years after December 31, 2012, the Reconciliation Act will a tax equal to 3.8% of the *lesser* of

- net investment income for such taxable year, or
- the excess of modified adjusted gross income (MAGI)[72] over $250,000 for joint filers ($125,000 for married filing separately and $200,000 for all other returns).

This tax is also applicable to income from estates and trusts. The active income from trade for self-employed and S-corporations will not be subject to the tax.[73] For these entities, the tax will apply only to passive income and trade income related to commodity trading. There is also a special provision for the application of the tax to S. Corporations which sell their businesses. *JCT estimates that this provision will increase revenues by $38.3 billion during FY2010-FY2014 and $210.2 billion during FY2010-FY2019.*

Appendix B. Timeline for Update Reductions Including Productivity Adjustments, by Provider Type

Table B-1. Timeline for Update Reductions Including Productivity Adjustments, by Provider

Provider	Productivity Adjustment	CY2009	CY2010	CY2011	CY2012	CY2013	CY2014	CY2015	CY2016	CY2017	CY2018
Acute care hospitals	October 1, 2011 Sec. 3401(a) of PPACA.	0.25 percentage points starting October 1, 2009. Sec. 3401(a) (effective April 1, 2010) Sec.3401(p) of PPACA.	0.25 percentage points starting October 1, 2010. Sec. 3401(a) of PPACA.	0.1 percentage point reduction in October 1, 2011. Sec.10319(a) of PPACA.	0.1 percentage points in October 1, 2012. Sec.10319(a) of PPACA.	0.3 percentage points in October 1, 2013. Sec. 1105(a) of the Reconciliation Act.	0.2 percentage points in October 1, 2014. Sec.1105(a) of HCERA.	0.2 percentage points in October 1, 2015. Sec. 1105(a) of HCERA.	0.75 percentage points in October 1, 2016. Sec. 1105(a) of HCERA.	0.75 percentage points in October 1, 2017. Sec. 1105(a) of HCERA.	0.75 percentage points in October 1, 2018. Sec. 1105(a) of HCERA.
Hospital outpatient departments	January 1, 2012. Sec. 3401(i) of PPACA.		0.25 percentage points starting January 1, 2010 Sec. 3401(i) of PPACA.	0.25 percentage point reduction in January 1, 2011 Sec. 3401(i) of PPACA.	0.1 percentage points in January 1, 2012 Sec. 10319(g) of PPACA.	0.1 percentage points in January 1, 2013. Sec. 10319(g) of PPACA.	0.3 percentage points in January 1, 2014 Sec. 1105(e) of HCERA.	0.2 percentage points in January 1, 2015. Sec. 1105(e) of HCERA.	0.2 percentage points in January 1, 2016. Sec. 1105(e) of HCERA.	0.75 percentage points in January 1, 2017. Se.c 1105(e) of HCERA.	0.75 percentage points in January 1, 2018,[a] **and January 1, 2019** Sec. 1105(e) of HCERA.
Inpatient psychiatric facilities	July 1, 2012. Sec. 3401(f) of PPACA.		0.25 percentage points starting July	0.25 percentage point reduction in July 1, 2011 Sec.10319(e) of PPACA.	0.1 percentage points in July 1, 2012 Sec.10319(e) of PPACA.	0.1 percentage points in July, 1, 2013 Sec 1105(d) of HCERA. 2 point reduction for no quality data starting July 1, 2013 Sec. 10322 of PPACA	0.3 percentage points in July 1, 2014. Sec. 1105(d) of HCERA.	0.2 percentage points in July 1, 2015 Sec. 1105(d) of HCERA.	0.2 percentage points in July 1, 2016 Sec. 1105(d) of HCERA.	0.75 percentage points in July 1, 2017 Sec. 1105(d) of HCERA.	0.75 percentage points in July 1, 2018,[b] and July 1, 2019 Sec. 1105(d) of HCERA.

Table B-1. (Continued)

Provider	Productivity Adjustment	CY2009	CY2010	CY2011	CY2012	CY2013	CY2014	CY2015	CY2016	CY2017	CY2018
Inpatient rehabilitation facilities	October 1, 2011. Sec. 3401(d) of PPACA.	0.25 percentage points starting October 1, 2009. Sec. 3401(d) (effective April 1, 2010) Sec. 3401(p) of PPACA.	0.25 percentage points starting October 1, 2010 Sec. 3401(d) of PPACA.	0.1percentage point reduction in October 1, 2011 Sec.10319(c) of PPACA.	0.1 percentage points in October 1, 2012 Sec.10319(c) of PPACA.	0.3 percentage points in October 1, 2013 Sec. 1105(c) of HCERA.	0.2 percentage points in October 1, 2014 Sec.1105(c) of HCERA.	0.2 percentage points in October 1, 2015 Sec. 1105(c) of HCERA.	0.75 percentage points in October 1, 2016 Sec. 1105(c) of HCERA.	0.75 percentage points in October 1, 2017 Sec. 1105(c) of HCERA.	0.75 percentage points in October 1, 2018 Sec. 1105(c) of HCERA.
Home health agencies	January 1, 2015. Sec. 3401(e) of PPACA.			1.0 percentage point reduction in January 1, 2011 Sec. 3401(e) of PPACA.	1.0 percentage point reduction in January 1, 2012 Sec. 3401(e) of PPACA.	1.0 percentage point reduction in January 1, 2013 Sec.10319(d) of PPACA.					
Skilled nursing homes	October 1, 2011. Sec. 3401(b) of PPACA.										
Long term care hospitals	October 1, 2011. Sec. 3401(c) of PPACA.	0.25 percentage points starting October 1, 2009. Sec. 3401(c) (effective April 1, 2010). Sec. 3401(p) of PPACA.	0.5 percentage points starting October 1, 2010 Sec. 0319(b) of PPACA.	0.1 percentage point reduction in October 1, 2011 Sec. 10319(b) of PPACA.	0.1 percentage points in October 1, 2012 Sec. 10319(b) of PPACA.	0.3 percentage points in October 1, 2013 Sec. 1105(b) of HCERA.	0.2 percentage points in October 1, 2014 Sec 1105(b) of HCERA.	0.2 percentage points in October 1, 2015. Sec. 1105(b) of HCERA.	0.75 percentage points in October 1, 2016. Sec. 1105(b) of HCERA.	0.75 percentage points in October 1, 2017. Sec. 1105(b) of HCERA.	0.75 percentage points in October 1, 2018. Sec. 1105(b) of HCERA
Hospice	October 1, 2012. Sec. 3401(g) of PPACA.				0.3 percentage points [from 0.5 by Sec. 10319(f)] in October 1, 2012	0.3 percentage points [from 0.5 by Sec. 10319(f)] in October 1, 2013 subject	0.3 percentage points [from 0.5 by Sec. 10319(f)] in October	0.3 percentage points [from 0.5 by Sec. 10319(f)] in October 1, 2015 subject	0.3 percentage points [from 0.5 by Sec. 10319(f)] in October 1, 2016 subject	0.3 percentage points [from 0.5 by Sec. 10319(f)] in October 1, 2017 subject	0.3 percentage points [from 0.5 by Sec. 10319(f)] in October 1, 2018 subject

Table B-1. (Continued)

Provider	Productivity Adjustment	CY2009	CY2010	CY2011	CY2012	CY2013	CY2014	CY2015	CY2016	CY2017	CY2018
			Sec. 3401(g) of PPACA.	to a change in the number of insured above a 5% threshold. Sec. 3401(g) of PPACA.	1, 2014 subject to a change in the number of insured above a 5% threshold. Sec. 3401(g) of PPACA.	to a change in the number of insured above a 5% threshold. Sec. 3401(g) of PPACA.	to a change in the number of insured above a 5% threshold. Sec.3401(g) of PPACA.	to a change in the number of insured above a 5% threshold. Sec. 3401(g) of PPACA.	to a change in the number of insured above a 5% threshold. Sec. 3401(g) of PPACA.		
Clinical laboratory services	January 1, 2011(Replaces existing reduction of 0.5% in CY 2011-CY2013) Sec. 3401(l) of PPACA.	1.75 percentage points in January 1, 2011. Sec. 3401(l) of PPACA.	1.75 percentage points in January 1, 2012. Sec. 3401(l) of PPACA.	1.75 percentage points in January 1, 2013. Sec. 3401(l) of PPACA.	1.75 percentage points in January 1, 2014. Sec. 3401(l) of PPACA.	1.75 percentage points in January 1, 2015. Sec. 3401(l) of PPACA.					
Dialysis	January 1, 2012. (Replaces existing reduction of 1.0 percentage point) Sec. 3401(h) of PPACA.										
Ambulance services	January 1, 2011. Sec. 3401(j) of PPACA										
ASCs	January 1, 2011. Sec. 3401(k) of PPACA.										
All other Part B providers	January 1, 2011. Sec. 3401(o) of PPACA.										

a. The hospital outpatient department payment update will also be reduced 0.75 percentage points starting January 1, 2019.

b. The inpatient psychiatric facility payment update will also be reduced 0.75 percentage points starting July 1, 2019

Appendix C. Implementation Timeline of Medicare Provisions in PPACA

Table C-1 through **Table C-12** list the start date, effective date, or deadline for the Medicare changes established by PPACA (P.L. 111-148, as amended by P.L. 111-152) in chronological order. Where applicable, the frequency, duration, and end date associated with specific changes or requirements are noted in a separate column. Provisions that had non-specific implementation requirements or deadlines are presented separately in **Table C-13.** For additional information on provisions that appear in the timeline, refer to the more detailed summaries in **Appendix A**.[74] For definitions of acronyms used in the timeline, refer to **Appendix D**.

Table C-1. Start Date, Effective Date, or Deadline—Prior to 2010

Prior to 2010						
PPACA (P.L. 111-148)	**PPACA Title 10**	**Reconciliation Act (P.L. 111-152)**	**Provision Title**	**Description**	**Start or Effective Date or Deadline**	**End Date, Frequency or Duration**
3128			Technical Correction Related to Critical Access Hospital Services.	Establishes Medicare payments for qualifying ambulance services provided by a CAH or by an entity owned and operated by a CAH at 101% of reasonable costs rather than 100%.	1/1/2004	
3137(a)	10317		Hospital Wage Index Improvement.	Extends Section 508 Classifications (for hospitals unable to otherwise qualify for administrative reclassification to areas with higher wage index values) through 9/30/2010.	10/1/2009	9/30/2010
6301	10602		Patient-Centered Outcomes Research.	$10 million transferred from Treasury to PCORTF for FY2010.	10/1/2009	9/30/2010

Table C-2. Start Date, Effective Date, or Deadline—CY2010

2010						
PPACA (P.L. 111-148)	**PPACA Title 10**	**Reconciliation Act (P.L. 111-152)**	**Provision Title**	**Description**	**Start or Effective Date or Deadline**	**End Date, Frequency or Duration**
2902			Elimination of Sunset For Reimbursement for All Medicare Part B Services Furnished By Certain Indian Hospitals and Clinics.	Requires Medicare Part B reimbursements for items and services furnished in, or at the direction of, facilities operated by the Indian Health Service, an Indian tribe or an Indian tribal organization. on January 1, 2010.	1/1/2010	All subsequent years.
3002	10327		Improvements to the Physician Quality Reporting System.	Successful reporting in 2010 creates eligibility for 1.0% bonus paid in 2011.	1/1/2010	12/31/2010
3027			Extension of Gainsharing Demonstration.	Duration of existing gainsharing projects extended from current termination date of 12/31/2009.	1/1/2010	9/30/2011
3102			Extension of the Work Geogra-phic Index Floor and Revisions to the Practice Expense Geographic Adjust-ment Under the Medicare Physician Fee Schedule.	Extends the 1.00 floor for the geographic index for physician work from prior termination date of 12/31/2009.	1/1/2010	12/31/2010
3102			Extension of the Work Geographic Index Floor and Revisions to the Practice Expense Geographic Adjust-ment Under the Medicare Physician Fee Schedule.	Secretary to adjust the practice expense GPCI for 2010 and 2011 to reflect 1/2 of the difference between the relative costs of employee wages and rents in each of the different fee schedule areas and the national averages.	1/1/2010	12/31/2011
3103			Extension of Exceptions Process for Medicare Therapy Caps.	Extends the exceptions process for therapy caps from prior expiration of	1/1/2010	12/31/2010

Table C-2. (Continued)

2010						
PPACA (P.L. 111-148)	**PPACA Title 10**	**Reconciliation Act (P.L. 111-152)**	**Provision Title**	**Description**	**Start or Effective Date or Deadline**	**End Date, Frequency or Duration**
				12/31/2009.		
3104			Extension of Payment for Technical Component of Certain Physician Pathology Services.	Direct payment for the technical component of certain pathology services is extended from prior expiration date of 12/31/2009.		
3105(a)	10311		Extension of Ambulance Add-ons.	Bonus payments and increased ground ambulance payments are extended from prior expiration date of 12/31/2009.	1/1/2010	1/1/2011
3105(b)	10311		Extension of Ambulance Add-ons.	Payment of certain urban air ambulance services as rural air ambulance services is extended from current expiration date of 12/31/2009,	1/1/2010	12/31/2010
3107			Extension of Physician Fee Schedule Mental Health Add-On.	Extends a 5% add-on payment for mental health services, from prior expiration date of 12/31/2009.	1/1/2010	12/31/2010
3111			Payment for Bone Density Tests.	Increases payments for DXA services in 2010 and 2011; payments set at 70% of the 2006 reimbursement rates.	1/1/2010	12/31/2011
3121			Extension and Expansion of Outpatient Hold Harmless Provision.	Rural hospitals (with no more than 100 beds) that are not SCHs are eligible for hold harmless payments of 85% of the prior HOPD payment amount. All SCHs will receive 85% HOPD hold harmless payments.	1/1/2010	12/31/2010

Table C-2. (Continued)

2010						
PPACA (P.L. 111-148)	**PPACA Title 10**	**Reconciliation Act (P.L. 111-152)**	**Provision Title**	**Description**	**Start or Effective Date or Deadline**	**End Date, Frequency or Duration**
3129			Extension of and Revisions to Medicare Rural Hospital Flexibility Program.	Establishes new uses for Medicare flex grants.	1/1/2010	All subsequent years.
		1109	Payment for Qualifying Hospitals.	Pay $400 million to IPPS hospitals in lowest quartile of counties according to age, sex and race adjusted Part A and B benefit payments per beneficiary.	1/1/2010	9/30/2012
3201	10318	1102(f)	Medicare Advantage Payment.	Repeal of Comparative Cost Adjustment Program	1/1/2010	
3205			Extension for Specialized MA Plans for Special Needs Individuals.	Temporarily extends SNP authority.	1/1/2010	12/31/2013
3205			Extension for Specialized MA Plans for Special Needs Individuals.	Extends period during which SNPs that do not have contracts with Medicaid programs may continue to operate, but not expand their service area.	1/1/2010	12/31/2012
3206			Extension of Reasonable Cost Contracts.	Extends for 3 years the time reasonable cost plans may operate regardless of other MA plans in the area.	1/1/2010	1/1/2013
3208			Making Senior Housing Facility Demonstration Permanent.	Secretary required to establish new MA plan allowed to limit service area to a senior housing facility.	1/1/2010	All subsequent years.
3301		1101	Medicare Coverage Gap Discount Program for Brand- Name Drugs and Closing the Medicare	Medicare Part D enrollees who reach the coverage gap in 2010 receive a $250 rebate.	1/1/2010	12/31/2010

Table C-2. (Continued)

2010						
PPACA (P.L. 111-148)	**PPACA Title 10**	**Reconciliation Act (P.L. 111-152)**	**Provision Title**	**Description**	**Start or Effective Date or Deadline**	**End Date, Frequency or Duration**
			Prescription Drug "Donut Hole."			
3401	10319	1105	Revision of Certain Market Basket Updates and Incorporation of Productivity Improvements into Market Basket Updates That Do Not Already Incorporate Such Improvements.	HOPD: CY2010 and CY2011 update reduction of 0.25 percentage points.	1/1/2010	12/31/2011
4105			Evidence-Based Coverage of Medicare Preventive Services.	Authorizes the Secretary to modify coverage of preventive services under Part B, including by with holding payment, as long as changes are consistent with recommendations of the U.S. Preventive Services Task Force	1/1/2010	All subsequent years.
6003			Disclosure Requirements for In-Office Ancillary Services Exception to the Prohibition on Physician Self-Referral for Certain Imaging Services.	With respect to MRI, CT, PET, and other services as determined by Secretary, referring physician must inform individual in writing at time of referral that individual may obtain services from someone other than referring physician in same group practice as referring physician, or indivi-dual supervised by referring physician or physician in group practice. A written list of area suppliers must be provided.	1/1/2010	All subsequent years.

Table C-2. (Continued)

2010						
PPACA (P.L. 111-148)	**PPACA Title 10**	**Reconciliation Act (P.L. 111-152)**	**Provision Title**	**Description**	**Start or Effective Date or Deadline**	**End Date, Frequency or Duration**
6404			Maximum Period of Submission of Medicare Claims Reduced to Not More Than 12 Months.	Secretary is required to reduce maximum period for submission of Medicare claims to no more than 12 months instead of 3 years.	1/1/2010	All subsequent years.
6406			Requirement for Physicians to Provide Documentation on Referrals to Programs at High Risk of Waste and Abuse.	Secretary has the authority to disenroll, for no more than one year, a Medicare enrolled physician or supplier that fails to maintain and provide access to written orders or requests for payment for DME, certification for home health services, or referrals for other items and services to the Secretary.	1/1/2010	All subsequent years.
6407	10605		Face-to-Face Encounter with Patient Required Before Physicians May Certify Eligibility for Home Health Services or Durable Medical Equipment Under Medicare.	Physicians required to have a face-to-face encounter (including through telehealth) with the individual prior to issuing a certification or re-certification for home health services or DME.	1/1/2010	All subsequent years.
6408			Enhanced Penalties.	Secretary has the authority to impose penalties on MA or Part D plans that commit certain marketing violations, including enrolling beneficiaries in a plan without their consent, transferring an individual from one plan to another for the purpose of earning a commission, failing to comply with	1/1/2010	All subsequent years.

Table C-2. (Continued)

2010						
PPACA (P.L. 111-148)	**PPACA Title 10**	**Reconciliation Act (P.L. 111-152)**	**Provision Title**	**Description**	**Start or Effective Date or Deadline**	**End Date, Frequency or Duration**
				marketing requirements, or employing or contrac-ting with an individual or entity that violates the terms of the contract.		
6408			Enhanced Penalties.	Secretary has the authority to impose a CMP in the amount of $50,000 on persons who knowingly make, use, or cause to be made or used any false statement material to a fraudulent claim.	1/1/2010	All subsequent years.
6408			Enhanced Penalties.	Secretary has the authority to impose a CMP of $15,000 on persons who fail to grant timely access, upon reasonable request to the OIG, for the purpose of audits, investigations, evaluations, or other statutory functions of the OIG for each day of failure.	1/1/2010	All subsequent years.
3109			Exemption of Certain Pharmacies from Accreditation Requirements	Upon enactment, delays accreditation requirement for all pharmacies, although all pharmacies must meet accreditation requirements to participate in competitive bidding.	3/23/2010	1/11/2011
3110			Part B Special Enrollment Period for Disabled Tricare Beneficiaries.	A 12-month special enrollment period is created so that military retirees eligible for TRICARE and entitled to Medicare Part A, who had previously	3/23/2010	All subsequent years.

Table C-2. (Continued)

2010						
PPACA (P.L. 111-148)	**PPACA Title 10**	**Reconciliation Act (P.L. 111-152)**	**Provision Title**	**Description**	**Start or Effective Date or Deadline**	**End Date, Frequency or Duration**
				declined Part B, may sign up for Part B without penalty during the 12-month period beginning on the day after the last day of the initial enrollment period of the individual or, if later, the 12-month period beginning with the month the individual is notified by the Secretary of Defense of enrollment.		
3112			Revision to the Medicare Improvement Fund.	Eliminates the funding in the MIF.	3/23/2010	
	10323		Medicare Coverage for Individuals Exposed to Environmental Health Hazards.	Certain individuals exposed to environmental hazards are eligible for medical coverage and medical screening services.	3/23/2010	
3123	10313		Extension and Expansion of Rural Community Hospital Demonstration Program.	Expansion of budget neutral demonstration project for additional qualifying rural hospitals.	3/23/2010	9/30/2015
3126			Improvements to the Demonstration Project on Community Health Integration Models in Certain Rural Counties.	Eliminates the limit of 6 eligible counties that may participate in the demonstration project within the qualifying states. Rural health clinic services no longer one of specified CAH services. Rural health clinic services removed from the definition of other essential services and replaced with physician services.	3/23/2010	All subsequent years.

Table C-2. (Continued)

3131	10315		Payment Adjustments for Home Health Care.	Reduces the standard HHRG payment amounts for home health agencies such that aggregate reduction will equal five percent of total prospective HH payments. Restricts the total amount of additional payments for outliers from exceeding 2.5% of total HH prospective payments in a given fiscal year (or calendar year). Implementation date for this provision was not specified.	3/23/2010	All subsequent years.
3134			Misvalued Codes Under the Physician Fee Schedule.	Secretary to periodically identify physician services as being potentially misvalued, and make appropriate adjustments to the relative values of such services under the Medicare physician fee schedule.	3/23/2010	All subsequent years.
3134			Misvalued Codes Under the Physician Fee Schedule.	Repeals Section 4505(d) of the Balanced Budget Act of 1997, which established requirements for developing new resource-based practice expense relative value units, as well as Section 1868(a) of the Social Security Act (42 U.S.C. 1395ee(a)), which established the Practicing Physicians Advisory Council, a group of physicians who meet quarterly to discuss proposed changes in regulations and carrier manual instructions related to physician services.	3/23/2010	

Table C-2. (Continued)

2010						
PPACA (P.L. 111-148)	**PPACA Title 10**	**Reconciliation Act (P.L. 111-152)**	**Provision Title**	**Description**	**Start or Effective Date or Deadline**	**End Date, Frequency or Duration**
	10327(c)		Elimination of MA Regional Plan Stabilization Fund.	Eliminates the MA regional plan stabilization fund and transfers amounts in the fund to the Part B trust fund.	3/23/2010	
3306			Funding Outreach and Assistance for Low-Income Programs.	Extends MIPPA Section 119 and provides an additional $45 million for outreach and education activities related to Medicare low-income assistance programs for FY2010-FY2012 and is available until expended.	3/23/2010	Until expended.
3311			Improved Medicare Prescription Drug Plan and MA-PD Complaint System.	The Secretary is to develop and maintain a system to handle complaints regarding Part D plans or their sponsors which has the ability to report and initiate appropriate interventions and monitoring and to guide quality improvement.	3/23/2010	All subsequent years.
6001	10601	1106	Limitation on Medicare Exception to the Prohibition on Certain Physician Referrals for Hospitals.	Precludes physician-owned ambulatory surgery centers from converting to a hospital and qualifying for exemption from the Stark self-referral prohibition after the date of enactment.	3/23/2010	All subsequent years.
6001	10601	1106	Limitation on Medicare Exception to the Prohibition on	Establishes that the percentage of the total value of the physician ownership	3/23/2010	All subsequent

Table C-2. (Continued)

2010						
PPACA (P.L. 111-148)	**PPACA Title 10**	**Reconciliation Act (P.L. 111-152)**	**Provision Title**	**Description**	**Start or Effective Date or Deadline**	**End Date, Frequency or Duration**
			Certain Physician Referrals for Hospitals.	or investment interest in the hospital or in an entity whose assets include the hospital cannot increase after the date of enactment.		years.
6301	10602		Patient-Centered Outcomes Research.	PCOR Trust Fund created.	3/23/2010	
6401	10603	1304	Provider Screening and Other Enrollment Requirements Under Medicare, Medicaid, and CHIP.	Providers or suppliers enrolling or re-enrolling in Medicare, Medicaid, or CHIP will be required to disclose current or previous affiliations with any provider or supplier that has uncollected debt, has had their payments suspended, has been excluded, or has had their billing privileges revoked.	3/23/2010	All Subsequent years.
6401	10603	1304	Provider Screening and Other Enrollment Requirements Under Medicare, Medicaid, and CHIP.	Medicare, Medicaid, and CHIP providers will be required to establish a compliance program, in accordance with requirements established by the Secretary.	3/23/2010	All subsequent years.
6402		1303	Enhanced Medicare and Medicaid Program Integrity Provisions.	CMS is to include in its IDR claims and payment data from the following programs: Medicare (Parts A, B, C, and D), Medicaid, CHIP, health-related programs administered by the VA and	3/23/2010	All subsequent years.

Table C-2. (Continued)

2010						
PPACA (P.L. 111-148)	**PPACA Title 10**	**Reconciliation Act (P.L. 111-152)**	**Provision Title**	**Description**	**Start or Effective Date or Deadline**	**End Date, Frequency or Duration**
				DOD, Social Security, and IHS. The Secretary is required to enter into data sharing agreements with the federal agencies above for the purposes of identifying fraud, waste, and abuse.		
6402		1303	Enhanced Medicare and Medicaid Program Integrity Provisions.	Secretary is required to impose penalties against beneficiaries entitled to or enrolled in Medicare, Medicaid, or CHIP who knowingly participate in a health care fraud offense.	3/23/2010	All subsequent years.
6402		1303	Enhanced Medicare and Medicaid Program Integrity Provisions.	Individuals required to report and return an overpayment within 60 days (instead of 30 days). Overpayments reported after this date will be considered an obligation as defined in Title 31 of the USC.	3/23/2010	All subsequent years.
6402		1303	Enhanced Medicare and Medicaid Program Integrity Provisions.	Individuals or entities that make a false statement or misrepresentation on an application to enroll or participate in a federal health care program are subject to OIG's permissive exclusion authority.	3/23/2010	All subsequent years.
6402		1303	Enhanced Medicare and Medicaid Program Integrity Provisions.	Secretary has the authority to impose a penalty in the amount of $50,000 on individuals who have been excluded	3/23/2010	All subsequent years.

Table C-2. (Continued)

2010						
PPACA (P.L. 111-148)	PPACA Title 10	Reconciliation Act (P.L. 111-152)	Provision Title	Description	Start or Effective Date or Deadline	End Date, Frequency or Duration
				from a federal health care program who order or prescribe an item or service; individuals who make false statements on enrollment applications, bids, or contracts to participate in a federal health care program; or persons who know of an overpayment and do not return the overpayment.		
6402		1303	Enhanced Medicare and Medicaid Program Integrity Provisions.	The Secretary has statutory authority to suspend payments to providers and suppliers pending an investigation of fraud.	3/23/2010	All Subsequent years.
6403			Elimination of Duplication Between the Healthcare Integrity and Protection Data Bank and the National Practitioner Data Bank.	The Secretary is required to begin implementing a transition process for transferring data stored in the HIPDB to the NPDB.	3/23/2010	
6411			Expansion of the Recovery Audit Contractor Program.	The Secretary is required to begin entering into contracts with RACs for Medicare Part C and D activities.	3/23/2010	12/31/2010
	10606		Health Care Fraud Enforcement.	The U.S. Sentencing Commission will now be required to review and amend the federal sentencing guidelines and policy statements applicable to persons convicted of federal health care offenses.	3/23/2010	

Table C-2. (Continued)

2010						
PPACA (P.L. 111-148)	**PPACA Title 10**	**Reconciliation Act (P.L. 111-152)**	**Provision Title**	**Description**	**Start or Effective Date or Deadline**	**End Date, Frequency or Duration**
	10606		Health Care Fraud Enforcement.	Certain existing criminal offenses are deemed as "federal healthcare fraud offenses" under the U.S. Criminal Code. Convictions for violations of the pecified statutes may be punishable by longer prison terms and/or higher fines, and other enforcement mechanisms may apply.	3/23/2010	
		1302	Medicare Prepayment Medical Review Limitations.	Medicare contractors no longer have to abide by limitations established in the MMA related to pre-payment review of claims.	3/23/2010	All subsequent years.
3131	10315		Payment Adjustments for Home Health Care.	Start date for rural add-on payments to HHAs.	4/1/2010	1/1/2016
3401	10319	1105	Revision of Certain Market Basket Updates and Incorporation of Productivity Improvements into Market Basket Updates That Do Not Already Incorporate Such Improvements.	IPPS hospital: FY2010 update reduction of 0.25 percentage points (applies to discharges beginning on the specified date).	4/1/2010	9/30/2010
3401	10319	1105	Revision of Certain Market Basket Updates and Incorporation of Productivity Improvements into Market Basket Updates That Do Not Already Incorporate Such	IRF: FY2010 update reduction of 0.25 percentage points (applies to discharges beginning on the specified date).	4/1/2010	9/30/2010

Table C-2. (Continued)

2010						
PPACA (P.L. 111-148)	**PPACA Title 10**	**Reconciliation Act (P.L. 111-152)**	**Provision Title**	**Description**	**Start or Effective Date or Deadline**	**End Date, Frequency or Duration**
			Improvements.			
3401	10319	1105	Revision of Certain Market Basket Updates and Incorporation of Productivity Improvements into Market Basket Updates That Do Not Already Incorporate Such Improvements.	LTCH: RY2010 update reduction of 0.25 percentage points (applies to discharges beginning on the specified date).	4/1/2010	9/30/2010
3122			Extension of Medicare Reason-able Costs Payments for Certain Clinical Diagnostic Laboratory Tests Furnished to Hospital Patients in Certain Rural Areas.	Cost reimbursement for clinical laboratory services provided by certain qualifying rural hospitals with less than 50 beds will be reinstated for one year.	7/1/2010	7/1/2011
3135		1107	Modification of Equipment Utilization Factor for Advanced Imaging Services.	Increase the technical component payment reduction for sequential imaging services on contiguous body parts during the same visit from 25% to 50%.	7/1/2010	All subsequent years.
3139			Payment for Biosimilar Biological Products.	A Part B biosimilar product approved by the FDA may be reimbursed at the ASP of the biosimilar plus 6% of the reference product.	7/1/2010	All subsequent years.
3401	10319	1105	Revision of Certain Market Basket Updates and Incorporation of Productivity Improvements into Market Basket Updates That	IPF: RY2011 and RY2012 update reduction of 0.25 percentage points.	7/1/2010	6/30/2012

Table C-2. (Continued)

2010						
PPACA (P.L. 111-148)	**PPACA Title 10**	**Reconciliation Act (P.L. 111-152)**	**Provision Title**	**Description**	**Start or Effective Date or Deadline**	**End Date, Frequency or Duration**
			Do Not Already Incorporate Such Improvements.			
6405	10604		Physicians Who Order Items and Services Required to be Medicare Enrolled Physicians or Eligible Professionals.	Deadline for physicians or eligible professionals who submit written orders or certifications for DME or HH services to be enrolled in the Medicare program.	7/1/2010	
6401	10603	1304	Provider Screening and Other Enrollment Requirements Under Medicare, Medicaid, and CHIP.	Secretary has 180 days to develop, in consultation with the OIG, procedures related to provider screening, Secretary has the authority to begin charging institutional providers $500 to cover the costs of the screening.	9/19/2010	
6301	10602		Patient-Centered Outcomes Research.	CG appoints 17 PCORI Board members.	9/23/2010	
6409			Medicare Self-Referral Disclosure Protocol.	Secretary, in cooperation with the OIG, must establish a SRDP to enable health care providers and suppliers to disclose actual or potential violations of the physician self-referral law. Secretary must also post information on CMS' website on how to disclose actual or potential SRDP violations.	9/23/2010	
3123	10313		Extension of the Rural Community Hospital	Extends budget neutral demonstration project for participating rural hospitals	10/1/2010	9/30/2015

Table C-2. (Continued)

2010						
PPACA (P.L. 111-148)	PPACA Title 10	Reconciliation Act (P.L. 111-152)	Provision Title	Description	Start or Effective Date or Deadline	End Date, Frequency or Duration
			Demonstration Program.	for an additional 5 years.		
3125	10314		Temporary Improvements to the Medicare Inpatient Hospital Payment Adjustment for Low-Volume Hospitals.	Eases the distance requirements (from a 25 to a 15 road mile separation), alters the number of discharges (from 800 total discharges to 1,600 Medicare discharges) and increases the percentage adjustment qualifying low volume hospitals (beginning FY 2011).	10/1/2010	10/1/2012
3128			Technical Correction Related to Critical Access Hospital Services.	Reinstates Medicare payments for certain HOPD facility services to 101% of reasonable costs.	10/1/2010	All subsequent years.
	10324		Protections for Frontier States.	Establish wage index floor of 1 for IPPS hospitals in certain frontier states	10/1/2010	All subsequent years.
3137	10317		Hospital Wage Index Improvement.	Restores reclassification thresholds (to be used by the MGCRB when making reclassification decisions) to the percentages used in FY2009 and in subsequent fiscal years until the first fiscal year that is one year after the date of submission of the Secretary's wage index reform plan. This date could be earlier if HHS submits report to Congress earlier than 12/31/2011.	10/1/2010	12/31/2012 or earlier
3141			Application of Budget Neutrality	Application of national budget	10/1/2010	All

Table C-2. (Continued)

2010						
PPACA (P.L. 111-148)	**PPACA Title 10**	**Reconciliation Act (P.L. 111-152)**	**Provision Title**	**Description**	**Start or Effective Date or Deadline**	**End Date, Frequency or Duration**
			on a National Basis in the Calculation of the Medicare Hospital Wage Index Floor for Each All-Urban and Rural State.	neutrality adjustment to adjust for the effect of the rural and imputed rural floor. This replaces the state budget neutrality adjustment that had begun to be phased in by CMS.		subsequent years.
	10325		Revision to Skilled Nursing Facility Prospective Payment System.	Secretary must implement change in final rule for FY2010 regarding concurrent therapy and changes to the lookback period.	10/1/2010	
3401	10319	1105	Revision of Certain Market Basket Updates and Incorporation of Productivity Improvements into Market Basket Updates That Do Not Already Incorporate Such Improvements.	IPPS hospital: FY2011 update reduction of 0.25 percentage points.	10/1/2010	9/30/2011
3401	10319	1105	Revision of Certain Market Basket Updates and Incorporation of Productivity Improvements into Market Basket Updates That Do Not Already Incorporate Such Improvements.	IRF: FY2011 update reduction of 0.25 percentage points.	10/1/2010	9/30/2011
3401	10319	1105	Revision of Certain Market Basket Updates and Incorporation of Productivity Improvements into Market Basket Updates That	LTCH: RY2011 update reduction of 0.5 percentage points.	10/1/2010	9/30/2011

Table C-2. (Continued)

2010						
PPACA (P.L. 111-148)	**PPACA Title 10**	**Reconciliation Act (P.L. 111-152)**	**Provision Title**	**Description**	**Start or Effective Date or Deadline**	**End Date, Frequency or Duration**
			Do Not Already Incorporate Such Improvements.			
6301	10602		Patient-Centered Outcomes Research.	$50 million transferred from Treasury to PCORTF for FY2011.	10/1/2010	9/30/2011
3142			HHS Study on Urban Medicare-Dependent Hospitals.	Secretary submits study and recommendations to Congress about increased payments to certain small urban Medicare dependent hospitals.	12/23/ 2010	
3106	10312		Extension of Certain Payment Rules for Long-term Care Hospital Services and of Moratorium on the Establishment of Certain Hospitals and Facilities.	The 3 year moratorium on the enforcement of certain LTCH payment rules and the establishment of new LTCHs is extended from 12/29/2010 for 2 years.	12/29/ 2010	12/29/2012
3137	10317		Hospital Wage Index Improvement.	Deadline by which CMS pays certain hospitals an additional amount to reflect the fact that those hospitals had a lower wage index from October 1, 2009, through March 31, 2010, than from April 1, 2010, through September 30, 2010, due to the temporary expiration of Section 508 reclassifications.	12/31/ 2010	
6001	10601	1106	Limitation on Medicare Exception to the Prohibition on Certain Physician Referrals for Hospitals.	Establishes that physician-owned hospitals that have provider agreements by this date and meet certain requirements will be exempt from the Stark self-referral prohibition.	12/31/ 2010	

Table C-3. Start Date, Effective Date, or Deadline—CY2011

2011						
PPACA (P.L. 111-148)	**PPACA Title 10**	**Reconciliation Act (P.L. 111-152)**	**Provision Title**	**Description**	**Start or Effective Date or Deadline**	**End Date, Frequency or Duration**
3002	10327		Improvements to the Physician Quality Reporting System.	Successful reporting of PQRI measures by physicians in 2011, 2012, and 2013 creates eligibility for 0.5% bonus for 2012, 2013, and 2014, respectively.	1/1/2011	12/31/2013
3002	10327		Improvements to the Physician Quality Reporting System.	For physicians who meet requirements for Maintenance of Certification Program during this time, an additional 0.5% bonus is available.	1/1/2011	12/31/2014
3006	10301		Plans for a Value-Based Purchasing Program for Skilled Nursing Facilities, Home Health Agencies, and Ambula-tory Surgical Centers.	Secretary submits to Congress plans to implement Medicare value-based purchasing programs for ASCs.	1/1/2011	
3021	10306		Establishment of Center for Medicare and Medicaid Innovation Within CMS.	The Secretary is required to establish a Center for Medicare and Medicaid Innovation (CMI) within CMS that will test innovative payment and service delivery models to reduce program expenditures under Medicare, Medicaid, and CHIP.	1/1/2011	
3026			Community-Based Care Transitions Program.	Secretary establishes a 5-year program in which eligible hospitals and community-based organizations are funded to provide transition services.	1/1/2011	12/31/2015

Table C-3. (Continued)

2011						
PPACA (P.L. 111-148)	**PPACA Title 10**	**Reconciliation Act (P.L. 111-152)**	**Provision Title**	**Description**	**Start or Effective Date or Deadline**	**End Date, Frequency or Duration**
3108			Permitting Physician Assistants to Order Post-Hospital Extended Care Services.	Physician assistants without employment relationships with a SNF may certify the need for post-hospital extended care services.	1/1/2011	All subsequent years.
3109			Exemption of Certain Pharmacies from Accreditation Requirements	Exempts certain pharmacies from Medicare's accreditation requirement, although all pharmacies must meet accreditation require-ments to participate in competitive bidding.	1/1/2011	All subsequent years.
3114			Improved Access for Certified Nurse-Midwife Services.	Increased payments for certified nurse-midwife services will be allowed—up to 100% of the amount provided to physicians for the same service.	1/1/2011	All subsequent years.
3127			MedPAC Study on Adequacy of Medicare Payments for Health Care Providers Serving in Rural Areas.	MedPAC study including recommendations due to Congress.	1/1/2011	
	10324		Protections for Frontier States.	Establish wage index floor of 1 for HOPD services provided by acute care hospitals and in certain frontier states.	1/1/2011	All subsequent years.
	10324		Protections for Frontier States.	Establish a floor on the practice expense component for physician services provided in certain frontier states.	1/1/2011	All subsequent years.
3131	10315		Payment Adjustments for Home Health Care.	Secretary establishes a provider-specific annual outlier cap of 10% of HHA revenues.	1/1/2011	All subsequent years.

Table C-3. (Continued)

2011						
PPACA (P.L. 111-148)	**PPACA Title 10**	**Reconciliation Act (P.L. 111-152)**	**Provision Title**	**Description**	**Start or Effective Date or Deadline**	**End Date, Frequency or Duration**
3132			Hospice Reform.	Secretary begins collecting additional data and information to revise hospice payments.	1/1/2011	All subsequent years.
3132			Hospice Reform.	Secretary requires, on and after this date, that hospice physicians or advance practice nurses have face-to-face encounters to determine continued eligibility prior to recertification.	1/1/2011	All subsequent years.
3135		1107	Modification of Equipment Utilization Factor for Advanced Imaging Services.	Changes the utilization rate assumption for calculating the payment for advanced imaging equipment from 50%, as assumed in prior years, to 75%.	1/1/2011	All subsequent years.
3136 (a)(1)			Revision of Payment for Power-Driven Wheelchairs.	Changes rental payments for power wheel-chairs from 10% to 15% of the purchase price for the first 3 months, and from 7.5% to 6% for the remaining 10 months.	1/1/2011	All subsequent years.
3136 (a)(2)			Revision of Payment for Power-Driven Wheelchairs.	Restricts lump-sum purchase option to complex, rehabilitative power wheelchairs.	1/1/2011	All subsequent years.
3138			Treatment of Certain Cancer Hospitals.	If outpatient costs incurred by IPPS-exempt cancer hospitals for drugs and biologics are determined to exceed those of other HOPDs, establishes an appropriate OPPS adjustment for cancer hospitals, which applies to services furnished on or after this date.	1/1/2011	
3201	10318	1102(b)	Medicare Advantage Payment.	Holds the 2011 MA benchmarks at the 2010 level.	1/1/2011	12/31/2011

Table C-3. (Continued)

2011						
PPACA (P.L. 111-148)	**PPACA Title 10**	**Reconciliation Act (P.L. 111-152)**	**Provision Title**	**Description**	**Start or Effective Date or Deadline**	**End Date, Frequency or Duration**
3201	10318	1102(e)	Medicare Advantage Payment.	Application of coding intensity adjustment.	1/1/2011	All subsequent years.
3202			Benefit Protection and Simplification.	First year MA plans are prohibited from charging cost - sharing above FFS amounts for certain services.	1/1/2011	All subsequent years.
3204			Simplification of Annual Beneficiary Election Periods.	First year beneficiaries are prohibited from switching MA plans or enrolling in MA plan from FFS Medicare after the start of the new benefit year.	1/1/2011	All subsequent years.
3205			Extension for Specialized MA Plans for Special Needs Individuals.	Secretary is required to establish a frailty payment adjustment, similar to PACE, for fully integrated dual- eligible SNPs.	1/1/2011	All subsequent years.
3205			Extension for Specialized MA Plans for Special Needs Individuals.	Requires the Secretary to periodically evaluate, revise, and publish MA risk adjust-ment payment methodologies and recalibrate payments for higher medical and care coordination costs for specified conditions.	1/1/2011	Periodically in subsequent years.
3207			Technical Correction to MA Private Fee-for-Service Plans.	Secretary is granted authority to waive certain network requirements for employer-based PFFS with enrollment as of 10/1/2009.	1/1/2011	All subsequent years.
3209			Authority to Deny Plan Bids.	Clarifies that Secretary is not required to accept any or every bid submitted by an MA or Part D plan.	1/1/2011	All subsequent years.
3301		1101	Medicare Coverage Gap Discount Program for	Medicare Part D enrollees in the coverage gap receive a 50% manufacturer discount off	1/1/2011	12/31/2011

Table C-3. (Continued)

2011						
PPACA (P.L. 111-148)	**PPACA Title 10**	**Reconciliation Act (P.L. 111-152)**	**Provision Title**	**Description**	**Start or Effective Date or Deadline**	**End Date, Frequency or Duration**
			Brand-Name Drugs and Closing the Medicare Prescription Drug "Donut Hole."	the price of brand name drugs, and receive a Medicare subsidy of 7% of the cost of generic drugs.		
3302			Improvement in Determination of Part D Low-Income Benchmark Premium.	The Medicare Advantage rebate amounts and performance bonus payments will be excluded from the MA-PDP premium bids when calculating the low-income subsidy benchmark amounts.	1/1/2011	All subsequent years.
3303			Voluntary De Minimus Policy for Subsidy Eligible Individuals Under Prescription Drug Plans and MA-PD Plans.	Plan sponsors who bid a nominal amount above the regional low-income subsidy benchmark will be allowed to absorb the cost of the difference in order to qualify as an LIS-eligible plan.	1/1/2011	All subsequent years.
3304			Special Rule for Widows and Widowers Regarding Eligibility for Low-Income Assistance.	A redetermination of low-income subsidy eligibility will be delayed for a year after the death of a spouse.	1/1/2011	All subsequent years.
3305			Improved Information for Subsidy Eligible Indivi-duals Reassigned to Prescription Drug Plans and MA-PD Plans.	For beneficiaries who are reassigned to new LIS plans, the Secretary is to transmit within 30 days of the reassignment, information to the beneficiary about formulary differences between the former plan and the new plan with respect to the beneficiary's drug regime.	1/1/2011	

Table C-3. (Continued)

2011						
PPACA (P.L. 111-148)	**PPACA Title 10**	**Reconciliation Act (P.L. 111-152)**	**Provision Title**	**Description**	**Start or Effective Date or Deadline**	**End Date, Frequency or Duration**
3307			Improving Formulary Requirements for Prescrip-tion Drug Plans and MA-PD Plans with Respect to Certain Categories or Classes of Drugs.	Drug plan sponsors will be required to include in their plans' formularies all drugs in classes identified as classes of clinical concern by the Secretary.	1/1/2011	All subsequent years.
3308			Reducing Part D Premium Subsidy for High-Income Beneficiaries.	Beneficiaries whose incomes exceed certain income thresholds will be required to pay higher premiums.	1/1/2011	All subsequent years.
	10331		Public Reporting of Performance Information.	The Secretary is required to develop a Physician Compare Internet website with information on physicians enrolled in the Medicare program.	1/1/2011	
3314			Including Costs Incurred By AIDS Drug Assistance Programs And Indian Health Service In Provid- ing Prescription Drugs Toward The Annual Out Of Pocket Threshold Under Part D.	Costs paid by the Indian Health Service or under an AIDS Drug Assistance Program will count toward a Part D enrollee's out-of-pocket threshold.	1/1/2011	All subsequent years.
3401	10319	1105	Revision of Certain Market Basket Updates	HHA: CY2011, CY2012, and CY2103 update reduction of 1.0 percentage point.	1/1/2011	12/31/2013

Table C-3. (Continued)

2011						
PPACA (P.L. 111-148)	**PPACA Title 10**	**Reconciliation Act (P.L. 111-152)**	**Provision Title**	**Description**	**Start or Effective Date or Deadline**	**End Date, Frequency or Duration**
			and Incorporation of Productivity Improvements into Market Basket Updates That Do Not Already Incorporate Such Improvements.			
3401	10319	1105	Revision of Certain Market Basket Updates and Incor-poration of Productivity Improvements into Market Basket Updates That Do Not Already Incorporate Such Improvements.	SNF: implement productivity adjustment.	10/1/2011	All subsequent years.
3401	10319	1105	Revision of Certain Market Basket Updates and Incor-poration of Productivity Improvements into Market Basket Updates That Do Not Already Incorporate Such Improvements.	Clinical lab: CY2011-CY2015 update reduction of 1.75 percentage points.	1/1/2011	12/31/2015

Table C-3. (Continued)

2011						
PPACA (P.L. 111-148)	**PPACA Title 10**	**Reconciliation Act (P.L. 111-152)**	**Provision Title**	**Description**	**Start or Effective Date or Deadline**	**End Date, Frequency or Duration**
3401	10319	1105	Revision of Certain Market Basket Updates and Incorporation of Produc-tivity Improvements into Market Basket Updates That Do Not Already Incorporate Such Improvements.	Ambulance services, ASCs, clinical labs, and all other Part B services: implement productivity adjustment.	1/1/2011	All subsequent years.
3402			Temporary Adjustment to the Calculation of Part B Premiums.	Freeze at the 2010 levels the income thresholds for determining beneficiaries subject to the income-related premium for the period of 2011 through 2019.	1/1/2011	12/31/2019
4103	10402 (b)		Medicare Coverage of Annual Wellness Visit Providing a Personalized Prevention Plan.	Coverage without cost-sharing required for an annual wellness visit and Personalized prevention plan for Part B enrollees.	1/1/2011	All subsequent years.
4104	10406		Removal of Barriers to Preventive Services in Medicare.	Cost-sharing eliminated for almost all preventive services covered under Part B (i.e., those services recommended for use by the U.S. Preventive Services Task Force).	1/1/2011	All subsequent years.
5501			Expanding Access to Primary Care Services and General Surgery Services.	A 10% bonus for select E&M and general surgery codes under the Medicare fee schedule for five years.	1/1/2011	12/31/2015

Table C-3. (Continued)

2011						
PPACA (P.L. 111-148)	**PPACA Title 10**	**Reconciliation Act (P.L. 111-152)**	**Provision Title**	**Description**	**Start or Effective Date or Deadline**	**End Date, Frequency or Duration**
	10501 (i)		Development and Implementation of Prospective Payment System for FQHCs.	Includes the new Medicare definition of preventive services as an FQHC service.	1/1/2011	
	10501 (i)		Development and Implementation of Prospective Payment System for FQHCs.	Requires FQHCs to submit necessary data to establish the PPS.	1/1/2011	
	10501 (i)(2)		FQHCs May Be Reimbursed for Medicare Covered Preventive Services.	Provides that FQHCs may be reimbursed for Medicare covered preventive services.	1/1/2011	All subsequent years.
6401	10603	1304	Provider Screening and Other Enrollment Requirements Under Medicare, Medicaid, and CHIP.	The Secretary is required to impose a 90-day period of enhanced oversight on DME suppliers initially enrolling in the program in instances when there is a significant risk of fraud.	1/1/2011	All subsequent years.
6402		1303	Enhanced Medicare and Medicaid Program Integrity Provisions.	Deadline for the Secretary to issue a regulation mandating that all Medicare and Medicaid providers include their NPI on all claims and enrollment applications.	1/1/2011	
6410 (a)			Adjustments to the Medicare Durable Medical Equipment, Prosthetics, Orthotics,	Expands the number of competitive bidding areas included in round 2 by 21 areas when round 2 is implemented in 2011 (not necessarily 1/1/2011).	1/1/2011	All subsequent years.

Table C-3. (Continued)

2011						
PPACA (P.L. 111-148)	**PPACA Title 10**	**Reconciliation Act (P.L. 111-152)**	**Provision Title**	**Description**	**Start or Effective Date or Deadline**	**End Date, Frequency or Duration**
			and Supplies Competitive Acquisition Program			
	10330		Modernizing Computer and Data Systems of CMS to Support Improvements in Care Delivery.	Deadline for the Secretary to post a plan on its website for modernizing the computer and data systems of CMS.	1/23/2011	
	10336		GAO Study and Report on Medicare Beneficiary Access to High-Quality Dialysis Services.	The Comptroller General is to submit a report on the impact on beneficiaries' access to quality ESRD services by including specified oral drugs in the ESRD bundled prospective payment system.	3/23/2011	
6401	10603	1304	Provider Screening and Other Enrollment Requirements Under Medicare, Medicaid, and CHIP.	Revised screening measures will apply to new providers and suppliers enrolling in Medicare, Medicaid, and CHIP.	3/23/2011	
3027			Extension of Gainsharing Demonstration.	The current due date of 12/1/2008 for required interim report on quality improvement and savings is extended.	3/31/2011	
		1301	Community Mental Health Centers.	CMHCs required to demonstrate that they provide at least 40% of their services to individuals not eligible for Medicare.	4/1/2011	
4204 (e)			Immunizations.	Deadline for submission of GAO report on access to Part D-funded immunizations among Medicare beneficiaries	6/1/2011	

Table C-3. (Continued)

2011						
PPACA (P.L. 111-148)	**PPACA Title 10**	**Reconciliation Act (P.L. 111-152)**	**Provision Title**	**Description**	**Start or Effective Date or Deadline**	**End Date, Frequency or Duration**
3113			Treatment of Certain Complex Diagnostic Laboratory Tests.	Demonstration project under Medicare Part B that will make separate payments to laboratories for complex diagnostic laboratory tests provided to Medicare beneficiaries.	7/1/2011	6/30/2013
3313			Office of the Inspector General Studies and Reports.	The Office of the Inspector General of HHS is to issue its first report on the extent to which drugs commonly used by dual eligibles are included on drug formularies (reports required annually thereafter).	7/1/2011	Annually.
3006	10301		Plans for a Value-Based Purchasing Program for Skilled Nursing Facilities, Home Health Agencies, and Ambulatory Surgical Centers.	Secretary is to submit plans to Congress to implement Medicare value-based purchasing for HHAs and SNFs.	10/1/2011	
3124			Extension of the Medicare Dependent Hospital Program.	Extends the Medicare dependent hospital program, which provides additional payments to certain small rural hospitals.	10/1/2011	10/1/2012
	10325		Revision to Skilled Nursing Facility Prospective Payment System.	Secretary may not implement RUG-IV changes published in FY2010 final rule until this date.	10/1/2011	
3313			Office of the Inspector General Studies and Reports.	The Office of the Inspector General of HHS is to issue a report that compares covered prescription drug prices under Medicare Part D to those negotiated by state Medicaid plans.	10/1/2011	

Table C-3. (Continued)

2011						
PPACA (P.L. 111-148)	**PPACA Title 10**	**Reconciliation Act (P.L. 111-152)**	**Provision Title**	**Description**	**Start or Effective Date or Deadline**	**End Date, Frequency or Duration**
3401	10319	1105	Revision of Certain Market Basket Updates and Incor-poration of Produc-tivity Improvements into Market Basket Updates That Do Not Already Incorporate Such Improvements.	IPPS hospital, IRF, and LTCH: implement productivity adjustment.	10/1/2011	All subsequent years.
3401	10319	1105	Revision of Certain Market Basket Updates and Incorporation of Productivity Improvements into Market Basket Updates That Do Not Already Incorporate Such Improvements.	IPPS hospital and IRF: FY2012 and FY2013 update reduction of 0.1 percentage points.	10/1/2011	9/30/2013
3401	10319	1105	Revision of Certain Market Basket Updates and Incor-poration of Productivity Improve-ments into Market Basket Updates That Do Not Already Incorporate Such Improvements.	LTCH: implement productivity adjustment.	10/1/2011	All subsequent years.

Table C-3. (Continued)

2011						
PPACA (P.L. 111-148)	**PPACA Title 10**	**Reconciliation Act (P.L. 111-152)**	**Provision Title**	**Description**	**Start or Effective Date or Deadline**	**End Date, Frequency or Duration**
3401	10319	1105	Revision of Certain Market Basket Updates and Incor-poration of Productivity Improvements into Market Basket Updates That Do Not Already Incorporate Such Improvements.	LTCH: RY2012 and RY2013 update reduction of 0.1 percentage points.	10/1/2011	9/30/2013
6301	10602		Patient-Centered Outcomes Research.	$150 million transferred from Treasury to PCORTF for FY2012.	10/1/2011	9/30/2012
3137(b)	10317		Hospital Wage Index Improvement.	Deadline for HHS Secretary report to Congress on reforming wage index.	12/31/2011	

Table C-4. Start Date, Effective Date, or Deadline—CY2012

2012						
PPACA (P.L. 111-148)	**PPACA Title 10**	**Reconciliation Act (P.L. 111-152)**	**Provision Title**	**Description**	**Start or Effective Date or Deadline**	**End Date, Frequency or Duration**
3003			Improvements to the Physician Feedback Program.	Secretary to provide comparative resou-rce use pattern reports to physicians.	1/1/2012	Allsubsequent years.
3003			Improvements to the Physician Feedback Program.	Secretary to develop episode grouper.	1/1/2012	

Table C-4. (Continued)

2012						
PPACA (P.L. 111-148)	**PPACA Title 10**	**Reconciliation Act (P.L. 111-152)**	**Provision Title**	**Description**	**Start or Effective Date or Deadline**	**End Date, Frequency or Duration**
3007			Value-Based Payment Modifier Under the Physician Fee Schedule.	Secretary to publish (1) specific measures of cost and quality, (2) specific dates for implementation, and (3) the proposed prospective performance period for a budget-neutral value-based payment modifier.	1/1/2012	
3008			Payment Adjustment for Conditions Acquired in Hospitals.	HHS study on extending HAC policy to other providers is due to Congress.	1/1/2012	
3022	10307		Medicare Shared Savings Program.	Secretary establishes a shared savings program in which eligible ACOs qualify for an annual incentive bonus if they achieve a threshold savings amount established for the three-year agreement period.	1/1/2012	All subsequent years.
3024			Independence at Home Demonstration Program.	Secretary establishes Medicare demonstration project to test the use of home-based primary care teams for certain chronically ill beneficiaries.	1/1/2012	
3102			Extension of the Work Geographic Index Floor and Revisions to the Practice Expense Geographic Adjustment Under the Medicare Physician Fee	Based on the Secretary's analysis and evaluation of current methods of establishing PE GPCI under the physician fee schedule, the Secretary will make appropriate adjustments (for 2012 and subsequent years) to the PE	1/1/2012	All subsequent years.

Table C-4. (Continued)

2012						
PPACA (P.L. 111-148)	**PPACA Title 10**	**Reconciliation Act (P.L. 111-152)**	**Provision Title**	**Description**	**Start or Effective Date or Deadline**	**End Date, Frequency or Duration**
			Schedule.	GPCI to ensure accurate geographic adjustments across payment areas.		
3201	10318	1102(b)	Medicare Advantage Payment.	Begin phase-in of calculation tying benchmarks to spending in FFS Medicare. (Phase-in to take 2-6 years.)	1/1/2012	1/1/2013
3201	10318	1102(c)	Medicare Advantage Payment.	In general, 1.5 percentage point benchmark bonus for quality MA plans (4 stars or more out of a 5 star quality scale). Double the bonus for quality plans in qualifying areas.	1/1/2012	12/31/2012
3201	10318	1102(d)	Medicare Advantage Payment.	3-year phase-in of rebate calculation based on plan quality: 4.5 stars or greater = 70% rebate; 3.5 stars but less than 4.5 stars = 65%; less than 3.5 stars = 50%.	1/1/2012	Fully phased in by 1/1/2015
3204			Simplification of Annual Beneficiary Election Periods.	MA and Part D annual coordinated election period changed to October 15 to December 7th each year (from November 15 to December 31).	1/1/2012	All subsequent years.
3205			Extension for Specialized MA Plans for Special Needs Individuals.	SNPs are required to be approved by the National Committee for Quality Assurance (NCQA) in order to serve targeted populations.	1/1/2012	All subsequent years.
3301		1101	Medicare Coverage Gap Discount Program for Brand-	Medicare Part D enrollees in the coverage gap receive a 50%	1/1/2012	12/31/2012

Table C-4. (Continued)

2012						
PPACA (P.L. 111-148)	**PPACA Title 10**	**Reconciliation Act (P.L. 111-152)**	**Provision Title**	**Description**	**Start or Effective Date or Deadline**	**End Date, Frequency or Duration**
			Name Drugs and Closing the Medicare Prescription Drug "Donut Hole."	manufacturer discount off the price of brand name drugs, and receive a Medicare subsidy of 14% of the cost of generic drugs.		
3309			Elimination of Cost Sharing for Certain Dual Eligible Individuals.	No earlier than this date, cost-sharing may be eliminated for low-income enrollees who receive care under a home and community based waiver who would otherwise require institutional care.	1/1/2012	All subsequent years.
3310			Reducing Wasteful Dispensing of Outpatient Prescription gs in Long-Term Drug Care Facilities Under Prescription Drug Plans and MA-PD Plans.	Part D sponsors will be required to employ utilization management techniques determined by the Secretary when dispensing medications to beneficiaries in long- term care facilities to reduce waste.	1/1/2012	All subsequent years.
3312			Uniform Exceptions and Appeals Process for Prescription Drug Plans and MA-PD Plans.	Part D plans will be required to use a single, uniform exceptions and appeals process.	1/1/2012	All subsequent years.
3401	10319	1105	Revision of Certain Market Basket Updates and Incorporation of Productivity Improvements into Market Basket Updates That Do Not	HOPD: implement productivity adjustment.	1/1/2012	All subsequent years.

Table C-4. (Continued)

2012						
PPACA (P.L. 111-148)	**PPACA Title 10**	**Reconciliation Act (P.L. 111-152)**	**Provision Title**	**Description**	**Start or Effective Date or Deadline**	**End Date, Frequency or Duration**
			Already Incorporate Such Improvements.			
3401	10319	1105	Revision of Certain Market Basket Updates and Incorporation of Productivity Improvements into Market Basket Updates That Do Not Already Incorporate Such Improvements.	HOPD: CY2012 and CY2013 update reduction of 0.1 percentage points.	1/1/2012	12/31/2013
3401	10319	1105	Revision of Certain Market Basket Updates and Incorporation of Productivity Improvements into Market Basket Updates That Do Not Already Incorporate Such Improvements.	Dialysis: implement productivity adjustment.	1/1/2012	All subsequent years.
6001	10601	1106	Limitation on Medicare Exception to the Prohibition on Certain Physician Referrals for Hospitals.	Requires that the regulations establishing the application process be implemented.	1/1/2012	
6001	10601	1106	Limitation on Medicare Exception to the Prohibition on Certain Physician Referrals for Hospitals.	Requires the application process to permit expansion of certain qualifying physician-owned hospitals be established.	2/1/2012	

Table C-4. (Continued)

2012						
PPACA (P.L. 111-148)	**PPACA Title 10**	**Reconciliation Act (P.L. 111-152)**	**Provision Title**	**Description**	**Start or Effective Date or Deadline**	**End Date, Frequency or Duration**
3001	10335		Hospital Value-Based Purchasing Program.	Requires a 3-year budget-neutral VBP demonstration projects for CAHs be established.	3/23/2012	3/23/2015
3001	10335		Hospital Value-Based Purchasing Program.	Requires a 3-year budget-neutral VBP demonstration projects for small volume IPPS hospitals be established.	3/23/2012	3/23/2015
6409			Medicare Self-Referral Disclosure Protocol.	Secretary must submit report to Congress, not later than 18 months after the date on which the SRDP is established (no later than 6 months after enactment),on implementation of this section.	3/23/2012	
6402		1303	Enhanced Medicare and Medicaid Program Integrity Provisions.	Beginning with FY2011, the Secretary is required to submit an annual report (not later than 180 days after the end of each fiscal year) to Congress on the effectiveness of Medicare Integrity Program (MIP) funds.	3/28/2012	All subsequent years.
6004			Prescription Drug Sample Transparency.	No later than April 1 of each year, drug manufacturers and authorized distri-butors of applicable drugs must submit to Secretary the identity and quantity of drug samples requested and distributed under Section 503 of the Prescription Drug Marketing Act of 1987.	4/1/2012	All subsequent years.

Table C-4. (Continued)

2012						
PPACA (P.L. 111-148)	**PPACA Title 10**	**Reconciliation Act (P.L. 111-152)**	**Provision Title**	**Description**	**Start or Effective Date or Deadline**	**End Date, Frequency or Duration**
6001	10601	1106	Limitation on Medicare Exception to the Prohibition on Certain Physician Referrals for Hospitals.	Requires that compliance audits for physician owned hospitals be established.	5/1/2012	
3401	10319	1105	Revision of Certain Market Basket Updates and Incorporation of Productivity Improvements into Market Basket Updates That Do Not Already Incorporate Such Improvements.	IPF: implement productivity adjustment.	7/1/2012	All subsequent years.
3401	10319	1105	Revision of Certain Market Basket Updates and Incorporation of Productivity Improvements into Market Basket Updates That Do Not Already Incorporate Such Improvements.	IPF: RY2013 and RY2014 update reduction of 0.1 percentage points.	7/1/2012	6/30/2014
3001	10335		Hospital Value-Based Purchasing Program.	1.0% penalty to base DRG payment amounts for discharges from IPPS hospitals that do not provide high quality care to Medicare beneficiaries as indicated by their performance on certain measures.	10/1/2012	9/30/2013

Table C-4. (Continued)

2012						
PPACA (P.L. 111-148)	**PPACA Title 10**	**Reconciliation Act (P.L. 111-152)**	**Provision Title**	**Description**	**Start or Effective Date or Deadline**	**End Date, Frequency or Duration**
3001	10335		Hospital Value-Based Purchasing Program.	Hospital quality reporting requirements are modified to incorporate risk adjustment and to the extent practicable measures would be endorsed by consensus organizations.	10/1/2012	
3004			Quality Reporting for Long-term Care Hospitals, Inpatient Rehabilitation Hospitals and Hospice Programs.	Applicable quality measures for RY2014 for LTCHS and FY2014 for IRFs and hospices must be published.	10/1/2012	
3005			Quality Reporting for PPS-Exempt Cancer Hospitals.	Starting FY2014, IPPS exempt cancer hospitals that do not submit required quality data will have their update reduced by 2 percentage points.	10/1/2012	All subsequent years.
3005			Quality Reporting for PPS-Exempt Cancer Hospitals.	Applicable quality measures for FY2014 for cancer hospitals must be published.	10/1/2012	
	10322		Quality Reporting for Psychiatric Hospitals.	Applicable quality measures for RY2014 for IPFs must be published.	10/1/2012	
3025 (a)	10309		Hospital Readmissions Reduction Program.	Starting for discharges on this date, the Secretary is to establish a hospital readmissions reduction program for certain potentially preventable Medicare inpatient hospital readmissions covering 3 conditions with high volume or high rate (or both).	10/1/2012	All subsequent years.

Table C-4. (Continued)

2012						
PPACA (P.L. 111-148)	**PPACA Title 10**	**Reconciliation Act (P.L. 111-152)**	**Provision Title**	**Description**	**Start or Effective Date or Deadline**	**End Date, Frequency or Duration**
3025 (a)	10309		Hospital Readmissions Reduction Program.	The floor adjustment factor for hospital discharges is 0.99. The greater of the floor adjustment factor or the excess readmissions ratio will be used to lower hospital discharge payments for hospitals with excess readmissions.	10/1/2012	9/30/2013
3401	10319	1105	Revision of Certain Market Basket Updates and Incorporation of Productivity Improvements into Market Basket Updates That Do Not Already Incorporate Such Improvements.	Hospice: implement productivity adjustment.	10/1/2012	All subsequent years.
3401	10319	1105	Revision of Certain Market Basket Updates and Incorporation of Productivity Improvements into Market Basket Updates That Do Not Already Incorporate Such Improvements.	Hospice: FY2013 update reduction of 0.3 percentage points.	10/1/2012	9/30/2013
6301	10602		Patient-Centered Outcomes Research.	Fees from insured (including self-insured) plans transferred to PCORTF: $1 per insured life in 2013, $2 (adjusted for inflation) per insured life in FY2014 through FY2019.	10/1/2012	9/30/2019

Table C-4. (Continued)

2012						
PPACA (P.L. 111-148)	**PPACA Title 10**	**Reconciliation Act (P.L. 111-152)**	**Provision Title**	**Description**	**Start or Effective Date or Deadline**	**End Date, Frequency or Duration**
6301	10602		Patient-Centered Outcomes Research.	Funds transferred from Medicare Trust Funds to PCORTF: $1 per insured life in 2013, $2 (adjusted for inflation) per insured life inFY2014 through FY2019.	10/1/2012	9/30/2019
3021	10306		Establishment of Center for Medicare and Medicaid Innovation Within CMS.	Beginning in 2012 (no date specified), the Secretary is required to submit a report to Congress at least every other year on CMI activities.	Unspecified date in 2012	Not less than once every other year.

Table C-5. Start Date, Effective Date, or Deadline—CY2013

2013						
PPACA (P.L. 111-148)	**PPACA Title 10**	**Reconciliation Act (P.L. 111-152)**	**Provision Title**	**Description**	**Start or Effective Date or Deadline**	**End Date, Frequency or Duration**
	10331		Public Reporting of Performance Information.	The Secretary is required to implement a plan for making publicly available information on physician performance through Physician Compare on the CMS website.	1/1/2013	
3023	10308		National Pilot Program on Payment Bundling.	Secretary establishes a 5-year pilot to coordinate care across a hospital episode (inpatient and post-hospital).	1/1/2013	12/31/ 2017
3201	10318	1102(c)	Medicare Advantage Payment.	In general, 3.0 percentage point benchmark bonus for quality MA plans (4 stars or more	1/1/2013	12/31/ 2013

Table C-5. (Continued)

2013						
PPACA (P.L. 111-148)	**PPACA Title 10**	**Reconciliation Act (P.L. 111-152)**	**Provision Title**	**Description**	**Start or Effective Date or Deadline**	**End Date, Frequency or Duration**
				out of a 5 star quality scale). Double the bonus for quality plans in qualifying areas.		
3205			Extension for Specialized MA Plans for Special Needs Individuals.	Secretary is required to establish a process to transition SNP beneficiaries that do not qualify as special needs individuals to FFS Medicare or other MA plans (non-SNP). Beneficiaries enrolled in specialized MA plans prior to 1/1/2010 are to be transitioned FFS Medicare or non-SNP MA plans by this date.	1/1/2013	
3301		1101	Medicare Coverage Gap Discount Program for Brand-Name Drugs and Closing the Medicare Prescription Drug "Donut Hole."	Medicare Part D enrollees in the coverage gap receive a 50% manufac-turer discount and a Medicare subsidy of 2.5% of the cost of brand name drugs, and receive a Medicare subsidy of 21% of the cost of generic drugs.	1/1/2013	12/31/2013
	10328		Improvement in Part D Medication Therapy Management Programs.	Part D sponsors will be required to include in their MTM programs an annual comprehensive medication review, furnished in person or using telehealth technologies, and provide follow-up interventions as warranted.	1/1/2013	All subsequent years.
	10501 (i)		Development and Implementation of Prospective Payment System for FQHCs.	Establishes a new PPS for FQHC services.	1/1/2013	

Table C-5. (Continued)

2013						
PPACA (P.L. 111-148)	**PPACA Title 10**	**Reconciliation Act (P.L. 111-152)**	**Provision Title**	**Description**	**Start or Effective Date or Deadline**	**End Date, Frequency or Duration**
9015	10906		Additional Hospital Insurance Tax on High-Income Taxpayers.	PPACA imposes an additional income tax of 0.9% on high- income workers on wages over $200,000 for single filers and $250,000 for joint filers. Revenues from this provision are transferred to the Medicare Hospital Insurance Trust Fund (Part A)	1/1/2013	All subsequent years.
		1402	Unearned Income Medicare Contribution.	PPACA imposes a new tax on net investment income for households with modified adjusted gross income over $200,000 single and $250,000 filing jointly.	1/1/2013	All subsequent years.
3027			Extension of Gainsharing Demonstration.	The due date of 5/1/2010 for the required final report is extended.	3/31/ 2013	
6002			Transparency Reports and Reporting of Physician Ownership or Investment Interests.	On this date and on the 90th day of each calendar year thereafter, covered drug, device, biological and medical supply manufacturers that make a payment or another transfer of value to a covered recipient must report specified information on those transactions to the Secretary of HHS.	3/31/ 2013	All subsequent years.
6002			Transparency Reports and Reporting of Physician Ownership or Investment Interests.	On this date and on the 90th day of each calendar year thereafter, manufacturers and group purchasing organizations must report to the Secretary of HHS certain information regarding an ownership or investment	3/31/ 2013	All subsequent years.

Table C-5. (Continued)

2013						
PPACA (P.L. 111-148)	**PPACA Title 10**	**Reconciliation Act (P.L. 111-152)**	**Provision Title**	**Description**	**Start or Effective Date or Deadline**	**End Date, Frequency or Duration**
				interest held by a physician (or an immediate family member) in the manufacturer or group purchasing organization during the preceding year.		
3403	10320		Independent Payment Advisory Board.	Chief Actuary of CMS submits determination of whether projected Medicare per capita growth rate for the implementation year (two years later) exceeds the projected Medicare per capita target growth rate for the implementation year; determination submitted annually thereafter.	4/30/ 2013	All subsequent years.
	10322		Quality Reporting for Psychiatric Hospitals.	Starting RY2014, IPFs that do not submit required quality data will have their update reduced by 2 percentage points.	7/1/2013	All subsequent years.
3403	10320		Independent Payment Advisory Board.	By this date, IPAB submits draft copy of proposal to the Secretary for Secretary's review and comment, and to MedPAC.	9/1/2013	All subsequent years (subject to certain conditions)
4202(b)			Medicare Demonstration: Promotion of Healthy Lifestyles.	Deadline for Secretary to submit report to Congress on required evaluation of community-based prevention and wellness programs that have demonstrated potential to help Medicare beneficiaries through	9/30/ 2013	

Table C-5. (Continued)

2013						
PPACA (P.L. 111-148)	**PPACA Title 10**	**Reconciliation Act (P.L. 111-152)**	**Provision Title**	**Description**	**Start or Effective Date or Deadline**	**End Date, Frequency or Duration**
				reducing their risk of disease, disability, and injury by making healthy lifestyle choices, including exercise, diet, and self-management of chronic diseases.		
3001	10335		Hospital Value-Based Purchasing Program.	1.25% penalty to base DRG payment amounts for discharges from IPPS hospitals that do not provide high quality care to Medicare beneficiaries as indicated by their performance on certain measures.	10/1/ 2013	9/30/2014
3001	10335		Hospital Value-Based Purchasing Program.	Hospital specific payments for MDHs would be subject to VBP penalty for discharges starting in FY2014 (such payments to SCHs are exempt in perpetuity).	10/1/ 2013	All subsequent years.
3004(a)			Quality Reporting for Long-term Care Hospitals, Inpatient Rehabilitation Hospitals and Hospice Programs.	Starting RY2014, LTCHs that do not submit required quality data will have their update reduced by 2 percentage points.	10/1/ 2013	All subsequent years.
3004(b)			Quality Reporting for Long-term Care Hospitals, Inpatient Rehabilitation Hospitals and Hospice Programs.	Starting FY2014, IRFs that do not submit required quality data will have their update reduced by 2 percentage points.	10/1/ 2013	All subsequent years.
3004(c)			Quality Reporting for Long-term Care Hospitals, Inpatient Rehabilitation Hospitals and Hospice Programs.	Starting FY2014, hospices that do not submit required quality data will have their update reduced by 2 percentage points.	10/1/ 2013	All subsequent years.

Table C-5. (Continued)

2013						
PPACA (P.L. 111-148)	**PPACA Title 10**	**Reconciliation Act (P.L. 111-152)**	**Provision Title**	**Description**	**Start or Effective Date or Deadline**	**End Date, Frequency or Duration**
3025(a)	10309		Hospital Readmissions Reduction Program.	The floor adjustment factor for hospital discharges is 0.98. The greater of the floor adjustment factor or the excess readmissions ratio will be used to lower hospital discharge payments for hospitals with excess readmissions.	10/1/ 2013	
3132			Hospice Reform.	Not earlier than this date, Secretary will implement budget neutral revisions to the hospice payment methodology.	10/1/ 2013	All subsequent years.
3133	10316	1041	Improvement to Medicare Disproportionate Share Hospital Payments.	Lowers Medicare DSH payments to IPPS hospitals to 25% of what otherwise would have been made.	10/1/ 2013	All subsequent years.
3133	10316	1041	Improvement to Medicare Disproportionate Share Hospital Payments.	Pays IPPS hospitals an additional amount that reflects (1) the difference in its DSH payments; (2) the difference in the uninsured minus 0.1 percentage points; and (3) the relative percentage of the hospital's uncompensated care.	10/1/ 2013	9/30/2014
3401	10319	1105	Revision of Certain Market Basket Updates and Incorporation of Productivity Improvements into Market Basket Updates That Do Not Already Incorporate Such Improvements.	IPPS hospital: FY2014 update reduction of 0.3 percentage points.	10/1/201 3	9/30/2014

Table C-5. (Continued)

2013						
PPACA (P.L. 111-148)	**PPACA Title 10**	**Reconciliation Act (P.L. 111-152)**	**Provision Title**	**Description**	**Start or Effective Date or Deadline**	**End Date, Frequency or Duration**
3401	10319	1105	Revision of Certain Market Basket Updates and Incorporation of Productivity Improvements into Market Basket Updates That Do Not Already Incorporate Such Improvements.	IRF: FY2014 update reduction of 0.3 percentage points.	10/1/2013	9/30/2014
3401	10319	1105	Revision of Certain Market Basket Updates and Incorporation of Productivity Improvements into Market Basket Updates That Do Not Already Incorporate Such Improvements.	LTCH: RY2014 update reduction of 0.3 percentage points.	10/1/2013	9/30/2014
3401	10319	1105	Revision of Certain Market Basket Updates and Incorporation of Productivity Improvements into Market Basket Updates That Do Not Already Incorporate Such Improvements.	Hospice: FY2014-FY2019 update reduction of 0.3 percentage points contingent on the level of the insured population relative to the projected insured population for the year preceding enactment (the level of the non-elderly insured population must be 5 or fewer percentage points above the projections for the update to take effect).	10/1/2013	9/30/2019
3007			Value-Based Payment Modifier Under the Physician Fee Schedule.	Secretary to begin implementing the value-based payment adjustment.	"2013 rulemaking process."	

Table C-6. Start Date, Effective Date, or Deadline—CY2014

2014						
PPACA (P.L. 111-148)	**PPACA Title 10**	**Reconciliation Act (P.L. 111-152)**	**Provision Title**	**Description**	**Start or Effective Date or Deadline**	**End Date, Frequency or Duration**
3007			Value-Based Payment Modifier Under the Physician Fee Schedule.	During performance period, Secretary is to provide information to physicians about the value of care they provide, as reflected by the measures of relative quality and cost.	1/1/2014	
3131	10315		Payment Adjustments for Home Health Care.	Secretary rebases home health payments. These adjustments are phased in over 4 years in equal increments that must not exceed 3.5% of the HH PPS base payment amount as of the date of enactment.	1/1/2014	12/31/2017
3133	10316	1041	Improvement to Medicare Disproportionate Share Hospital Payments.	Pays IPPS hospitals an additional amount that reflects (1) the difference in its DSH payments; (2) the difference in the uninsured minus 0.2 percentage points and (3) the relative percentage of the hospital's uncompensated care.	10/1/ 2014	9/30/2019
3201	10318	1102(c)	Medicare Advantage Payment.	In general, 5.0 percentage point benchmark bonus for quality MA plans (4 stars or more out of a 5 star quality scale). Double the bonus for quality plans in qualifying areas.	1/1/2014	All subsequent years.
3201	10318	1102 (e)	Medicare Advantage Payment.	Start of minimum required coding intensity adjustment of 1.3 percentage points above the 2010 adjustment, unless Secretary implements risk adjustment based on MA diagnostic, cost, and use data.	1/1/2014	All subsequent years.

Table C-6. (Continued)

2014						
PPACA (P.L. 111-148)	**PPACA Title 10**	**Reconciliation Act (P.L. 111-152)**	**Provision Title**	**Description**	**Start or Effective Date or Deadline**	**End Date, Frequency or Duration**
		1103	Savings from Limits on MA Plan Administrative Costs.	MA plans required to have a MLR of at least .85 or pay a fee. Restrict enrollment after 3 years of MLR below .85; terminate after 5 years.	1/1/2014	All subsequent years.
3301		1101	Medicare Coverage Gap Discount Program for Brand-Name Drugs and Closing the Medicare Prescription Drug "Donut Hole."	Medicare Part D enrollees in the cove-rage gap receive a Medicare subsidy of 2.5% and a 50% manufacturer discount on the cost of brand name drugs, and receive a Medicare subsidy of 28% of the cost of generic drugs; growth of true out-of-pocket expenses reduced by 0.25%.	1/1/2014	12/31/2014
3401	10319	1105	Revision of Certain Market Basket Updates and Incor-poration of Productivity Improve-ments into Market Basket Updates That Do Not Already Incorporate Such Improvements.	HOPD: CY2014 update reduction of 0.3 percentage points.	1/1/2014	12/31/2014
3403	10320		Independent Payment Advisory Board.	Board is required to submit its first proposal to the President and Congress if the projected Medicare per capita growth rate for the imple-mentation year exceeds the target growth rate for the implementation year. If the Medicare per capita growth rate does not exceed the target growth rate, the Board is required to submit an annual advisory report to Congress on matters related to the Medicare program.	1/15/ 2014	All subsequent years (subject to certain conditions).

Table C-6. (Continued)

2014						
PPACA (P.L. 111-148)	**PPACA Title 10**	**Reconciliation Act (P.L. 111-152)**	**Provision Title**	**Description**	**Start or Effective Date or Deadline**	**End Date, Frequency or Duration**
3403	10320		Independent Payment Advisory Board.	If Board fails to submit proposal to Congress and the President, Secretary submits contingent proposal.	1/25/2014	Each subsequent year (subject to certain conditions).
3131	10315		Payment Adjustments for Home Health Care.	Secretary submits a report to Congress on HHA costs associated with providing ongoing access to care to low-income Medicare beneficiaries or those in medically underserved areas, among other things.	3/1/2014	
3403	10320		Independent Payment Advisory Board.	Secretary submits report to Congress on results of review of Board's proposal (unless Secretary submits a proposal in that year). MedPAC submits comments to Congress on Board's proposal or the Secretary's proposal.	3/1/2014	All subsequent years (subject to certain conditions).
3403	10320		Independent Payment Advisory Board.	Deadline for specified Congressional Committees to consider the Board's proposal and report out legislative language implementing the recommendations. Congress has the authority to develop its own proposal provided it meets the same fiscal requirements as established for the Board.	4/1/2014	All subsequent years (subject to certain conditions).
3401	10319	1105	Revision of Certain Market Basket Updates and Incorporation of	IPF: RY2015 update reduction of 0.3 percentage points.	7/1/2014	6/30/2015

Table C-6. (Continued)

2014						
PPACA (P.L. 111-148)	**PPACA Title 10**	**Reconciliation Act (P.L. 111-152)**	**Provision Title**	**Description**	**Start or Effective Date or Deadline**	**End Date, Frequency or Duration**
			Productivity Improvements into Market Basket Updates That Do Not Already Incorporate Such Improvements.			
3403	10320		Independent Payment Advisory Board.	Deadline for the Board to produce a public report containing standardized information on system-wide health care costs, patient access to care, utilization, and quality of care that allows for comparison by region, types of services, types of providers, and both private and public payers. Report is to be produced annually thereafter.	7/1/2014	All subsequent years.
3403	10320		Independent Payment Advisory Board.	Start date for the Secretary to begin implementing the Board's proposal. Any recommendation that would change a provider's payment rate will apply to items and services furnished on the first day of the first fiscal year, calendar year, or rate year (which varies depending on provider type) that begins after August 15.	8/15/ 2014	Each subsequent year (subject to certain conditions).
3001	10335		Hospital Value-Based Purchasing Program.	1.5% penalty to base DRG payment amounts for discharges from IPPS hospitals that do not provide high quality care to Medicare beneficiaries as indicated by their performance on certain measures.	10/1/ 2014	9/30/2015

Table C-6. (Continued)

2014						
PPACA (P.L. 111-148)	**PPACA Title 10**	**Reconciliation Act (P.L. 111-152)**	**Provision Title**	**Description**	**Start or Effective Date or Deadline**	**End Date, Frequency or Duration**
3008			Payment Adjustment for Conditions Acquired in Hospitals.	IPPS hospitals in the top quartile of all IPPS hospitals as ranked by rates of HACs will have applicable payments reduced by 1.0%.	10/1/ 2014	All subsequent years.
3025(a)	10309		Hospital Readmissions Reduction Program.	The floor adjustment factor for hospital discharges is 0.97 for FY2015 and beyond. The greater of the floor adjustment factor or the excess readmissions ratio will be used to lower hospital discharge payments for hospitals with excess readmissions.	10/1/ 2014	All subsequent years.
3025(a)	10309		Hospital Readmissions Reduction Program.	Secretary expands the number of applicable procedures or conditions that are part of the hospital readmissions reduction program.	10/1/ 2014	All subsequent years.
3131	10315		Payment Adjustments for Home Health Care.	Secretary transfers $500 million for FY2015 through FY2018 for study and the home health care payment adjustment demonstration.	10/1/ 2014	9/30/2018
3401	10319	1105	Revision of Certain Market BasketUpdates and Incor-poration of Productivity Improvements into Market Basket Updates That Do Not Already Incorporate Such Improvements.	IPPS hospital: FY2015 and FY2016 update reduction of 0.2 percentage points.	10/1/ 2014	9/30/2016
3401	10319	1105	Revision of Certain Market Basket Updates and Incorporation of	IRF:FY2015 and FY2016 update reduction of 0.2 percentage points.	10/1/ 2014	9/30/2016

Table C-6. (Continued)

2014						
PPACA (P.L. 111-148)	**PPACA Title 10**	**Reconciliation Act (P.L. 111-152)**	**Provision Title**	**Description**	**Start or Effective Date or Deadline**	**End Date, Frequency or Duration**
			Productivity Improvements into Market Basket Updates That Do Not Already Incorporate Such Improvements.			
3401	10319	1105	Revision of Certain Market Basket Updates and Incorporation of Productivity Improvements into Market Basket Updates That Do Not Already Incorporate Such Improvements.	LTCH: RY2015 and RY2016 update reduction of 0.2 percentage points.	10/1/ 2014	9/30/2016

Table C-7. Start Date, Effective Date, or Deadline—CY2015

2015						
PPACA (P.L. 111-148)	**PPACA Title 10**	**Reconciliation Act (P.L. 111-152)**	**Provision Title**	**Description**	**Start or Effective Date or Deadline**	**End Date, Frequency or Duration**
3002	10327		Improvements to the Physician Quality Reporting System.	For physicians who do not report quality measures during this time, there is a penalty of 1.5% of Medicare Part B allowed charges.	1/1/2015	12/31/2015
3007			Value-Based Payment	Secretary to apply the payment modifier for	1/1/2015	All

Table C-7. (Continued)

2015						
PPACA (P.L. 111-148)	**PPACA Title 10**	**Reconciliation Act (P.L. 111-152)**	**Provision Title**	**Description**	**Start or Effective Date or Deadline**	**End Date, Frequency or Duration**
			Modifier Under the Physician Fee Schedule.	items and services furnished for specific physicians and groups of physicians the Secretary determines appropriate.		subsequent years.
	10331		Public Reporting of Performance Information.	The Secretary is required to submit to Congress a report on the Physician Compare Internet website.	1/1/2015	
3131	10315		Payment Adjustments for Home Health Care.	Taking into account the results of the study due March 1, 2014, the Secretary may conduct a 4- year demonstration testing whether HH payment adjustments would improve access for patients with high severity of illness or low income, or underserved patients. The demonstration would begin not later than this date.	1/1/2015	12/31/2018
3131	10315		Payment Adjustments for Home Health Care.	MedPAC submits a report to Congress on implementation of home health payment rebasing adjustments.	1/1/2015	
3201	10318	1102(e)	Medicare Advantage Payment.	Minimum required coding intensity adjustment of 0.25 percentage points above previous year's adjustment, unless Secretary implements risk adjustment based on MA diagnostic, cost, and use data.	1/1/2015	12/31/2015
3210			Development of New Standards for Certain Medigap Plans.	The National Association of Insurance Commissioners to create new model plans for Medigap C and F. To the extent	1/1/2015	

Table C-7. (Continued)

2015						
PPACA (P.L. 111-148)	**PPACA Title 10**	**Reconciliation Act (P.L. 111-152)**	**Provision Title**	**Description**	**Start or Effective Date or Deadline**	**End Date, Frequency or Duration**
				practicable, the revised standards for benefit packages will be implemented as of this date.		
3301		1101	Medicare Coverage Gap Discount Program for Brand-Name Drugs and Closing the Medicare Prescription Drug "Donut Hole."	Medicare Part D enrollees in the coverage gap receive a Medicare subsidy of 5% and a 50% manufacturer discount on the cost of brand name drugs, and receive a Medicare subsidy of 35% of the cost of generic drugs; growth of TrOOP expenses reduced by 0.25%.	1/1/2015	12/31/2015
3401	10319	1105	Revision of Certain Market Basket Updates and Incorporation of Productivity Improvements into Market Basket Updates That Do Not Already Incorporate Such Improvements.	HOPD: CY2015 and CY2016 update reduction of 0.2 percentage points.	1/1/2015	12/31/2016
3401	10319	1105	Revision of Certain Market Basket Updates and Incorporation of Productivity Improvements into Market Basket Updates That Do Not Already Incorporate Such Improvements.	HHA: implement productivity adjustment.	1/1/2015	All subsequent years.
3403	10320		Independent Payment Advisory Board.	Deadline for the Board to submit to Congress and the President advisory recommendations	1/15/2015	At least once every

Table C-7. (Continued)

2015						
PPACA (P.L. 111-148)	**PPACA Title 10**	**Reconciliation Act (P.L. 111-152)**	**Provision Title**	**Description**	**Start or Effective Date or Deadline**	**End Date, Frequency or Duration**
				to slow the rate of growth in NHE. These recommendations could not target expenditures in federal health care programs. Recommendations are required at a minimum once every two years.		2 years thereafter.
3113			Treatment of Certain Complex Diagnostic Laboratory Tests.	Secretary to submit assessment report on the 2- year demonstration project (begun on July 1, 2011) and recommendations to Congress.	6/30/2015	
3401	10319	1105	Revision of Certain Market Basket Updates and Incorporation of Productivity Improvements into Market Basket Updates That Do Not Already Incorporate Such Improvements.	IPF: RY2016 and RY2017 update reduction of 0.2 percentage points.	7/1/2015	6/30/2017
3403	10320		Independent Payment Advisory Board.	Due date for GAO report on changes to payment policies, methodologies, and rates resulting from the Board's recommendations.	7/1/2015	Periodically in subse-quent years.
3001	10335		Hospital Value-Based Purchasing Program.	1.75% penalty to base DRG payment amounts for discharges from IPPS hospitals that do not provide high quality care to Medicare beneficiaries as indicated by their performance on certain measures	10/1/2015	9/30/2016
3001	10335		Hospital Value-Based Purchasing Program.	Interim report from GAO on VBP program is due to Congress.	10/1/2015	

Table C-8. Start Date, Effective Date, or Deadline—CY2016

2016						
PPACA (P.L. 111-148)	**PPACA Title 10**	**Reconciliation Act (P.L. 111-152)**	**Provision Title**	**Description**	**Start or Effective Date or Deadline**	**End Date, Frequency or Duration**
3001	10335		Hospital Value-Based Purchasing Program.	HHS study on VBP program is due to Congress.	1/1/2016	
3002	10327		Improvements to the Physician Quality Reporting System.	Penalty of 2% of Part B charges for physicians who do not report quality measures.	1/1/2016	All subsequent years.
	10326		Pilot Testing Pay-For-Performance Programs for Certain Medicare Providers.	VBP pilot programs for IPFs, LTCHs, IRFs, IPPS exempt cancer hospitals, and hospice programs are implemented on a budget neutral basis. Subject to certain certifications by OACT, the Secretary would be able to expand the pilot projects after 1/1/2018.	1/1/2016	
3023	10308		National Pilot Program on Payment Bundling.	Secretary may expand the program after this date.	1/1/2016	
3201	10318	1102(e)	Medicare Advantage Payment.	Minimum required coding intensity adjustment of 0.25 percentage points above previous year's adjustment, unless Secretary implements risk adjustment based on MA diagnostic, cost, and use data.	1/1/2016	12/31/2016
3301		1101	Medicare Coverage Gap Discount Program for Brand-Name Drugs and Closing the	Medicare Part D enrollees in the coverage gap receive a Medicare subsidy of 5% and a 50% manufacturer discount on the cost of brand name drugs; and	1/1/2016	12/31/2016

Table C-8. (Continued)

2016						
PPACA (P.L. 111-148)	**PPACA Title 10**	**Reconciliation Act (P.L. 111-152)**	**Provision Title**	**Description**	**Start or Effective Date or Deadline**	**End Date, Frequency or Duration**
			Medicare Prescription Drug "Donut Hole."	receive a Medicare subsidy of 42% of the cost of generic drugs, growth in true out-of-pocket costs indexed to the lower of the original annual percentage increase of drug expenditures or CPI-Urban plus 2%.		
6410(b)			Adjustments to the Medicare Durable Medical Equipment, Prosthetics, Orthotics, and Supplies Competitive Acquisition Program.	Requires the Secretary to extend the Competitive Acquisition Program or apply competitively bid rates to remaining areas.	1/1/2016	All subsequent years.
3001	10335		Hospital Value-Based Purchasing Program.	HHS evaluation of VBP demonstration project for CAHs is due to Congress no later than 18 months from completion of the VBP demonstration project in CAHs.	9/23/2016	
3001	10335		Hospital Value-Based Purchasing Program.	HHS evaluation of VBP demonstration project for small volume IPPS hospitals is due to Congress no later than 18 months from completion of those VBP demonstration projects.	9/23/2016	
3001	10335		Hospital Value-Based Purchasing Program.	2.0% penalty to base DRG payment amounts for discharges from IPPS hospitals that do not provide high quality care to Medicare beneficiaries as indicated by their performance on certain measures.	10/1/2016	All subsequent years.

Table C-8. (Continued)

2016						
PPACA (P.L. 111-148)	**PPAC A Title 10**	**Reconciliation Act (P.L. 111-152)**	**Provision Title**	**Description**	**Start or Effective Date or Deadline**	**End Date, Frequency or Duration**
3401	10319	1105	Revision of Certain Market Basket Updates and Incorporation of Productivity Improve-ments into Market Basket Updates That Do Not Already Incorporate Such Improvements.	IPPS hospital: FY2017, FY2018, and FY2019 update reduction of 0.75 percentage points.	10/1/2016	9/30/2019
3401	10319	1105	Revision of Certain Market Basket Updates and Incorporation of Productivity Improvements into Market Basket Updates That Do Not Already Incorporate Such Improvements.	IRF: FY2017, FY2018, and FY2019 update reduction of 0.75 percentage points.	10/1/2016	9/30/2019
3401	10319	1105	Revision of Certain Market Basket Updates and Incorporation of Productivity Improvements into Market Basket Updates That Do Not Already Incorporate Such Improvements.	LTCH: RY2017, FY2018, and RY2019 update reduction of 0.75 percentage points	10/1/2016	9/30/2019

Table C-9. Start Date, Effective Date, or Deadline—CY2017

2017						
PPACA (P.L. 111-148)	**PPACA Title 10**	**Reconciliation Act (P.L. 111-152)**	**Provision Title**	**Description**	**Start or Effective Date or Deadline**	**End Date, Frequency or Duration**
3007			Value-Based Payment Modifier Under the Physician Fee Schedule.	Secretary to apply the payment modifier for items and services furnished for all physicians and groups of physicians.	1/1/2017	All subsequent years.
3133	10316	1041	Improvement to Medicare Disproportionate Share Hospital Payments.	Uses data from the Census Bureau as certified by OACT for certain aspects of the formula for hospitals' additional payments.	1/1/2017	All subsequent years.
3201	10318	1102(e)	Medicare Advantage Payment.	Minimum required coding intensity adjustment of 0.25 percentage points above previous year's adjustment, unless Secretary implements risk adjustment based on MA diagnostic, cost, and use data.	1/1/2017	12/31/2017
3301		1101	Medicare Coverage Gap Discount Program for Brand-Name Drugs and Closing the Medicare Prescription Drug "Donut Hole."	Medicare Part D enrollees in the coverage gap receive a Medicare subsidy of 10% and a 50% manufacturer discount on the cost of brand name drugs; and receive a Medicare subsidy of 49% of the cost of generic drugs, growth in true out-of-pocket costs indexed to the lower of the original annual percentage increase of drug expenditures or CPI- Urban plus 2%.	1/1/2017	12/31/2017
3401	10319	1105	Revision of Certain Market Basket Updates and Incorporation of Productivity	HOPD: CY2017, CY2018, and CY2019 update reduction of 0.75 percentage points.	1/1/2017	12/31/2019

Table C-9. (Continued)

2017						
PPACA (P.L. 111-148)	**PPACA Title 10**	**Reconciliation Act (P.L. 111-152)**	**Provision Title**	**Description**	**Start or Effective Date or Deadline**	**End Date, Frequency or Duration**
			Improvements into Market Basket Updates That Do Not Already Incorporate Such Improvements.			
3403	10320		Independent Payment Advisory Board.	Deadline for Congress to introduce a joint resolution discontinuing the Board's activities.	2/1/2017	
3001	10335		Hospital Value-Based Purchasing Program.	Final report from GAO on VBP program is due to Congress.	7/1/2017	
3401	10319	1105	Revision of Certain Market Basket Updates and Incorporation of Productivity Improvements into Market Basket Updates That Do Not Already Incorporate Such Improvements.	IPF: RY2018, RY2019, and RY2020 update reduction of 0.75 percentage points.	7/1/2017	6/30/2020
3403	10320		Independent Payment Advisory Board.	Deadline for Congress to enact a joint resolution discontinuing the Board's activities.	8/15/2017	

Table C-10. Start Date, Effective Date, or Deadline—CY2018

2018						
PPACA (P.L. 111-148)	**PPACA Title 10**	**Reconciliation Act (P.L. 111-152)**	**Provision Title**	**Description**	**Start or Effective Date or Deadline**	**End Date, Frequency or Duration**
3201	10318	1102 (e)	Medicare Advantage Payment.	Minimum required coding intensity adjustment of 0.25 percentage points above previous year's adjustment, unless Secretary implements risk adjustment based on MA diagnostic, cost, and use data.	1/1/2018	12/31/2018
3301		1101	Medicare Coverage Gap Discount Program for Brand-Name Drugs and Closing the Medicare Prescription Drug "Donut Hole."	Medicare Part D enrollees in the coverage gap receive a Medicare subsidy of 15% and a 50% manufacturer discount on the cost of brand name drugs; and receive a Medicare subsidy of 56% of the cost of generic drugs, growth in true out-of-pocket costs indexed to the lower of the original annual percentage increase of drug expenditures or CPI- Urban plus 2%.	1/1/2018	12/31/2018
3403	10320		Independent Payment Advisory Board.	Board is only required to submit proposals to the President and Congress for years in which the projected rate of growth in Medicare spending exceeds the Gross Domestic Product (GDP) plus 1.0%.	1/15/2018	All subsequent years.
6301	10602		Patient-Centered Outcomes Research.	CG review of the adequacy and use of the funding for the Institute.	3/23/2018	

Table C-11. Start Date, Effective Date, or Deadline—CY2019

2019						
PPACA (P.L. 111-148)	PPACA Title 10	Reconciliation Act (P.L. 111-152)	Provision Title	Description	Start or Effective Date or Deadline	End Date, Frequency or Duration
3201	10318	1102(e)	Medicare Advantage Payment.	Minimum required coding intensity adjustment of not less than 5.7 percent.	1/1/2019	All subsequent years.
3301		1101	Medicare Coverage Gap Discount Program for Brand-Name Drugs and Closing the Medicare Prescription Drug "Donut Hole."	Medicare Part D enrollees in the coverage gap receive a Medicare subsidy of 20% and a 50% manufacturer discount on the cost of brand name drugs; and receive a Medicare subsidy of 63% of the cost of generic drugs, growth in true out-of-pocket costs indexed to the lower of the original annual percentage increase of drug expenditures or CPI-Urban plus 2%.	1/1/2019	12/31/2019
3403	10320		Independent Payment Advisory Board.	The first year the Board may begin submitting proposals that may reduce payments to providers and suppliers scheduled to receive a reduction in their payment updates in excess of a reduction due to productivity. These proposals would take effect in 2020.	1/15/ 2019	All subsequent years.

Table C-12. Start Date, Effective Date, or Deadline—CY2020

2020						
PPACA (P.L. 111-148)	PPACA Title 10	Reconciliation Act (P.L. 111-152)	Provision Title	Description	Start or Effective Date or Deadline	End Date, Frequency or Duration
3301		1101	Medicare Coverage Gap Discount Program for Brand-Name Drugs and Closing the Medicare Prescription Drug "Donut Hole."	Medicare Part D enrollees in the coverage gap receive a Medicare subsidy of 25% and a 50% manufacturer discount on the cost of brand name drugs, and receive a Medicare subsidy of 75% of the cost of generic drugs; true out-of-pocket costs determined as if the 2014- 2019 adjustments had not been made.	1/1/2020	All subsequent years.

Table C-13. Unspecified Start Date, Effective Date, or Deadline

Unspecified						
PPACA (P.L. 111-148)	**PPACA Title 10**	**Reconciliation Act (P.L. 111-152)**	**Provision Title**	**Description**	**Start or Effective Date or Deadline**	**End Date, Frequency or Duration**
6301	10602		Patient-Centered Outcomes Research.	Methodology Committee to submit (1) methodological standards and (2) translation table for guidance to the PCORI Board.	18 months after establishment of the Institute.	
3023	10308		National Pilot Program on Payment Bundling.	Secretary submits interim report to Congress.	Not later than 2 years after implementation of pilot project	
3023	10308		National Pilot Program on Payment Bundling.	Secretary submits final report to Congress.	Not later than 3 years after implementation of pilot project.	
3111			Payment for Bone Density Tests.	Secretary to arrange with the IOM to study and report to the Secretary and Congress on the ramifications of Medicare reimbursement reductions for DXA on beneficiary access to bone mass measurement benefits.	Report due as provided in agreement between Secretary and IOM.	
6005			Pharmacy Benefit Managers Transparency Requirements.	Pharmacy Benefit Managers that contract with Part D drug plans or qualified health plans must share certain financial information with the Secretary of HHS, the plans the PBMs contract with through Medicare Part D, or the exchanges in a manner, form and timeframe specified by the Secretary.	To be determined by the Secretary.	

Table C-13. (Continued)

Unspecified						
PPACA (P.L. 111-148)	**PPACA Title 10**	**Reconciliation Act (P.L. 111-152)**	**Provision Title**	**Description**	**Start or Effective Date or Deadline**	**End Date, Frequency or Duration**
3024			Independence at Home Demonstration Program.	Secretary submits a final report to Congress with an analysis of the demonstration project on coordination of care, expendi-tures, access to care, and quality of care.	Unspecified.	
3140			Medicare Hospice Concurrent Care Demonstration Program.	Secretary conducts a 3-year demonstration to allow hospice patients to receive all other Medicare covered services.	Unspecified.	
3140			Medicare Hospice Concurrent Care Demonstration Program.	Secretary conducts independent evaluation of the demonstration program and submits report to Congress containing the results of the evaluation.	Unspecified.	
3311			Improved Medicare Prescription Drug Plan and MA-PD Complaint System.	The Secretary must submit annual reports on the complaint system regarding Part D plans or their sponsors.	Unspecified.	All subsequent years.
6301	10602		Patient-Centered Outcomes Research.	PCORI incorporated.	Unspecified.	
6301	10602		Patient-Centered Outcomes Research.	CG appoints 15 methodology committee members.	Unspecified.	
6301	10602		Patient-Centered Outcomes Research.	Methodology Committee report to PCORI Board. PCORI annual report to Congress and the President.	Unspecified.	
6301	10602		Patient-Centered Outcomes Research.	Contract for annual financial audit of the PCORI.	Unspecified.	

Table C-13. (Continued)

Unspecified						
PPACA (P.L. 111-148)	**PPACA Title 10**	**Reconciliation Act (P.L. 111-152)**	**Provision Title**	**Description**	**Start or Effective Date or Deadline**	**End Date, Frequency or Duration**
6301	10602		Patient-Centered Outcomes Research.	CG review of the annual financial audits of the PCORI.	Unspecified.	All subsequent years.
6301	10602		Patient-Centered Outcomes Research.	CG review of the processes of the PCORI for objectivity and credibility.	Unspecified.	Every 5 years.
6301	10602		Patient-Centered Outcomes Research.	CG review of the dissemination and training activities and data networks established by the PCORI.	Unspecified.	Every 5 years.
6301	10602		Patient-Centered Outcomes Research.	CG review of the overall effectiveness of activities of the PCORI.	Unspecified.	Every 5 years.
	10323		Medicare Coverage for Individuals Exposed to Environmental Health Hazards.	The Secretary is required to establish a pilot program, with appropriate reimbursement methodologies, to provide comprehensive, coordinated, and cost-effective care to certain individuals who enroll in Part B and who are diagnosed with an illness caused by an environmental hazard to which an EPA emergency declaration applies.	Unspecified.	
6301	10602		Patient-Centered Outcomes Research.	CG annual report to Congress on results of reviews done that year. Due April 1st of each year (does not specify year of first due date).	April 1, first year unspecified	All subsequent years.

Appendix D. List of Acronyms

ACO	Accountable Care Organization
ASC	Ambulatory Surgery Center
ASP	Average Sales Price
CY	Calendar Year
CAH	Critical Access Hospital
CG	Comptroller General (of the Government Accountability Office)
CHIP	State Children's Health Insurance Program
CMI	Center for Medicare and Medicaid Innovation
CMP	Civil Monetary Penalty
CMS	Centers for Medicare & Medicaid Services
DGME	Direct Graduate Medical Education
DOD	Department of Defense
DRG	Diagnostic Related Group
DSH	Disproportionate Share Hospital
DXA	Dual Energy X-Ray Absorptiometry
E&M	Evaluation and Management
FFS	Fee-for-Service
FQHC	Federally Qualified Health Center
FY	Fiscal Year
GAO	Government Accountability Office
GPCI	Geographic Practice Cost Indices
HAC	Hospital Acquired Condition
HHA	Home Health Agency
HHRG	Home Health Resource Group
HHS	U.S. Department of Health and Human Services
HIPD	Healthcare Integrity and Protection Data Bank
HOPD	Hospital Outpatient Department
IDR	Integrated Data Repository
IHS	Indian Health Services
IME	Indirect Medical Education
IOM	Institute of Medicine
IPF	Inpatient Psychiatric Facility
IPPS	Inpatient Prospective Payment System
IRF	Inpatient Rehabilitation Facility
LIS	Low Income Subsidy
LTCH	Long Term Care Hospital
MA	Medicare Advantage
MA-PDP	Medicare Advantage Prescription Drug Plan
MDH	Medicare Dependent Hospital
MedPAC	Medicare Payment Advisory Commission
MGCRB	Medicare Geographic Classification Review Board
MIF	Medicare Improvement Fund

MIPPA	Medicare Improvements for Patients and Providers Act (P.L. 110-275; enacted July 15, 2008)
MTM	Medication Therapy Management
NPDB	National Practitioner Data Bank
OACT	Office of the Actuary of CMS
OIG	Office of Inspector General of HHS
PBM	Pharmacy Benefit Manager
PCOR	Patient-Centered Outcomes Research
PCORI	Patient-Centered Outcomes Research Institute
PCORTF	Patient-Centered Outcomes Research Trust Fund
PE GPCI	Practice Expense Geographic Practice Cost Indices
PFFS	Private Fee for Service
PPS	Prospective Payment System
PQRI	Physician Quality Reporting Initiative
RAC	Recovery Audit Contractors
RY	Rate Year
SCH	Sole Community Hospital
Secretary	Secretary of the Department of Health and Human Services
SNF	Skilled Nursing Facility
SNP	Special Needs Plans
SRDP	Self-Referral Disclosure Protocol
USC	United States Code
VA	Departments of Veterans Affairs
VBP	Value-Based Purchasing

Acknowledgments

Cliff Binder, Christopher Davis, Sarah Lister, Janemarie Mulvey, Kirsten Colello, Amanda Sarata, Jennifer Staman, and Holly Stockdale also contributed to this report.

End Notes

[1] CBO's Baseline Projections of Medicare Spending, March 2009, http://www.cbo.gov/budget/factsheets/2009b/medicare.pdf.

[2] Those provisions are discussed in CRS Report R40943, *Public Health, Workforce, Quality, and Related Provisions in the Patient Protection and Affordable Care Act (P.L. 111-148)*, coordinated by C. Stephen Redhead and Erin D. Williams.

[3] Background information on the Medicare program can be found in the CRS Report R40425, *Medicare Primer*.

[4] The CBO score on PPACA combined with the Reconciliation Act, may be found at http://www.cbo.gov/ftpdocs/113xx/doc11379/Manager'sAmendmenttoReconciliationProposal.pdf. The JCT score may be found at http://www.jct.gov/publications.html?func=startdown&id=3672.

[5] The estimated overall effect of the proposed legislation is a net decrease in the federal budget deficit of $143 billion over the FY2010-FY2019 period. The projected 10-year cost of increasing insurance coverage of $788 billion is offset by the net spending decrease of $511 billion and by revenue provisions that are estimated to raise $420 billion over the same period.

[6] CRS analysis of CBO March 20, 2010, estimates of the effects of PPACA and the Reconciliation Act combined (http://www.cbo.gov/ftpdocs/113xx/doc11379/Manager'sAmendmenttoReconciliationProposal.pdf).

[7] CBO expenditure projections for PPACA do not include all of the discretionary costs associated with the legislation. CBO expects Department of Health and Human Services costs to increase at least $5 billion to $10 billion over 10 years.

[8] This estimate excludes interaction effects including the impact on these reductions to payments to Medicare Advantage plans and on the collection of Part B premiums.

[9] December 19, 2009, CBO analysis of Senate H.R. 3590; http://www.cbo.gov/ftpdocs/108xx/doc10868/12-19-Reid_Letter_Managers_Correction_Noted.pdf.

[10] Subsequent to CBO's March 20, 2010, estimate, Congress has taken action several times to delay these payment reductions. For more detail on the SGR system and recent legislation affecting Medicare physician payments, see CRS Report R40907, *Medicare Physician Payment Updates and the Sustainable Growth Rate (SGR) System*, by Jim Hahn.

[11] In an April 22, 2010, report, "Estimated Financial Effects of the Patient Protection and Affordable Care Act, as Amended," the CMS Office of the Actuary (OACT) suggests that long-term savings from the productivity adjustments may be unrealistic. OACT estimates that approximately 15% of Part A providers could become unprofitable within the 10-year projection period as a result of productivity adjustments, and may therefore opt to end their participation in Medicare.

[12] Part A, the Hospital Insurance program, covers hospital services, up to 100 days of post-hospital skilled nursing facility services, post-institutional home health visits, and hospice services. Part B, the Supplementary Medical Insurance program, covers a broad range of medical services including physician services, laboratory services, durable medical equipment, and outpatient hospital services. Part B also covers some home health visits. Part C provides private plan options, such as managed care, for beneficiaries who are enrolled in both Parts A and B. Part D provides optional outpatient prescription drug coverage.

[13] Medicare has specific rules for fee-for-service payments under Parts A and B as well as capitation (or per person) payments under Part C. Outpatient prescription drugs covered under Part D are not subject to Medicare payment rules. Prices are determined through negotiation between prescription drug plans (PDPs), or Medicare Advantage Prescription Drug (MA-PD) plans, and drug manufacturers. The Secretary of Health and Human Services is statutorily prohibited from intervening in Part D drug price negotiations.

[14] Medicare Payment Advisory Commission (MedPAC) *Report to Congress: Medicare Payment Policy*, March 2009, http://www.medpac.gov/documents/Mar09_EntireReport.pdf.

[15] See pp. 35-41 of Medicare Payment Advisory Commission (MedPAC) *Report to Congress: Medicare Payment Policy*, March 2009, for a discussion of their update framework.

[16] The cost estimate issued by the CMS Office of the Actuary for PPACA, mentioned earlier, breaks down the savings associated with the changes to the update factors to different providers. According to their estimate, the market basket revisions for acute care hospitals including incorporation of the productivity adjustment in Section 3401 will save $112.6 billion over 10 years.

[17] Medicare Payment Advisory Commission (MedPAC) *Report to Congress: Medicare Payment Policy*, March 2007, pp. 70-87, http://www.medpac.gov/documents/Mar07_EntireReport.pdf.

[18] MedPAC's *March 2009 Report*, Section 2D, pp. 157-182.

[19] Centers for Medicare and Medicaid Services, "Medicare Program; Prospective Payment System and Consolidated Billing for Skilled Nursing Facilities for FY 2010; Minimum Data Set, Version 3.0 for Skilled Nursing Facilities and Medicaid Nursing Facilities," 74 *Federal Register* 153, August 11, 2009.

[20] H.R. 4213, as passed by the House of Representatives on May 28, 2010, would repeal this provision.

[21] Department of Health and Human Services, Centers for Medicare and Medicaid Services, "Medicare Program: Home Health Prospective Payment System Rate Update," 74 *Federal Register* 58077, November 10, 2009.

[22] Letter from Amy Hall, Office of Legislation, Centers for Medicare and Medicaid Services, U.S. House and Senate Notification, March 31, 2010.

[23] See CBO, "Comparison of Projected Enrollment in Medicare Advantage Plans and Subsidies for Extra Benefits Not Covered by Medicare Under Current Law and Under Reconciliation Legislation Combined with H.R. 3590 as Passed by Senate, March 19, 2010," at http://www.cbo.gov/ftpdocs/113xx/doc11355/MAComparisons.pdf.

[24] This estimate also includes the repeal of the Comparative Cost Adjustment program explained in detail in Appendix A.

[25] See CBO, "Comparison of Projected Enrollment in Medicare Advantage Plans and Subsidies for Extra Benefits Not Covered by Medicare Under Current Law and Under Reconciliation Legislation Combined with H.R. 3590 as Passed by Senate," March 19, 2010, http://www.cbo.gov/ftpdocs/113xx/doc11355/MAComparisons.pdf.

[26] MedPAC's *Report to Congress: Improving Incentives in the Medicare Program*, June 2009, http://www.medpac.gov/ documents/Jun09_EntireReport.pdf.

[27] Defined as groups of providers and suppliers who work together to manage and coordinate care for Medicare fee-for-service beneficiaries and who meet certain criteria specified by the Secretary.

[28] For additional information on Medicare financing see CRS Report RS20173, *Medicare: Financing the Part A Hospital Insurance Program*, by Patricia A. Davis, and CRS Report RS20946, *Medicare: History of Part A Trust Fund Insolvency Projections*, by Patricia A. Davis.

[29] 2009 Annual Report of the Boards of Trustees of the Federal Hospital Insurance and Federal Supplementary Medical Insurance Trust Funds, http://www.cms.hhs.gov/reportstrustfunds/.

[30] For beneficiaries enrolled in MA, Part C payments are made on their behalf in appropriate portions from the HI and SMI trust funds.

[31] CBO letter to Sen. Jeff Sessions, January 22, 2010, http://www.cbo.gov/ftpdocs/110xx/doc11005/01-22-HI_Fund.pdf. This estimate does not include the financial impact of changes made by the Reconciliation Act.

[32] CBO Report, "Estimated Effect of the Patient Protection and Affordable Care Act (Incorporating the Manager's Amendment) on the Hospital Insurance Trust Fund," December 23, 2009, http://www.cbo.gov/ftpdocs/108xx/doc10868/12-23-HI_TF_memo.pdf.

[33] CMS Office of the Actuary, "Estimated Effects of the Patient Protection and Affordable Care Act, as Amended, on the Year of Exhaustion for the Part A Trust Fund, Part B premiums, and Part A and B Coinsurance Amounts," April 22, 2010.

[34] The National Health Care Anti-Fraud Association (NHCAA) estimates conservatively that 3% of all health care spending—or $68 billion—is lost to health care fraud. See "The Problem of Health Care Fraud," available at http://www.nhcaa.org/eweb/DynamicPage.aspx?webcode=anti_fraud_resource_centr&wpscode=TheProblem OfHCFraud. The Federal Bureau of Investigation (FBI) estimates that as much as 10% of total health care expenditures could be lost to public and private sector health care fraud. See "Financial Crimes Report to the Public for Fiscal Year 2007," available at http://www.fbi.gov/publications/financial/fcs_report2007/financial_crime_2007.htm#health.

[35] Congressional Budget Office, "The Long-Term Budget Outlook," June 2009, pp. 9-10, http://www. cbo.gov/ftpd ocs/ 102xx/doc10297/06-25-LTBO.pdf.

[36] CBO estimate of the effects of PPACA and the Reconciliation Act, March 20, 2010, http://www.cbo.gov/ftpdocs/113xx/doc11379/Manager'sAmendmenttoReconciliationProposal.pdf, p. 14; and CMS Office of the Actuary, "Estimated Financial Effects of the Patient Protection and Affordable Care Act, as Amended," April 22, 2010.

[37] In addition, Sec. 3013(b) as modified by Sec. 10303(b) requires the Secretary to the extent practicable, to publicly report on measures for hospital-acquired conditions that are currently used by CMS for the adjustment of payment to hospitals based on rates of hospital-acquired infections.

[38] Provisions in Part II of Subtitle A of Title III, National Strategy to Improve Health Care Quality, and related Title X provisions are discussed in CRS Report R40943, *Public Health, Workforce, Quality, and Related Provisions in the Patient Protection and Affordable Care Act (P.L. 111-148)*, coordinated by C. Stephen Redhead and Erin D. Williams.

[39] See CRS Report R40907, *Medicare Physician Payment Updates and the Sustainable Growth Rate (SGR) System*, by Jim Hahn.

[40] H.R. 4213, as passed by the House of Representatives on May 28, 2010, would repeal this provision.

[41] In a separate score of the potential effects of PPACA on discretionary spending, CBO estimated that this provision would cost a total of $87 million for years 2011 and 2012 combined. Letter from Douglas W. Elmendorf to the Honorable Jerry Lewis, May, 11, 2010, http://www.cbo.gov/ftpdocs/114xx/ doc11490/LewisLtr_HR3590.pdf.

[42] H.R. 4213, as passed by the House of Representatives on May 28, 2010, would extend Section 508 reclassifications for an additional year, until September 30, 2011.

[43] Sections 7001-7003 in Subtitle A of Title VII on biologic price competition and innovation are discussed in CRS Report R40943, *Public Health, Workforce, Quality, and Related Provisions in the Patient Protection and Affordable Care Act (P.L. 111-148)*, coordinated by C. Stephen Redhead and Erin D. Williams.

[44] H.R. 4213, as passed by the House of Representatives on May 28, 2010, would repeal this provision.

[45] Centers for Medicare and Medicaid Services, "Medicare Program; Prospective Payment System and Consolidated Billing for Skilled Nursing Facilities for FY 2010; Minimum Data Set, Version 3.0 for Skilled Nursing Facilities and Medicaid Nursing Facilities," 74 *Federal Register* 153, August 11, 2009.

[46] Under the PACE program, Medicare contracts with organizations to provide comprehensive medical and social services to the frail elderly who enroll in the program. PACE plans, like MA plans, are paid on a capitated basis.

[47] MA plans with low enrollment may not have enough enrollees to either generate the quality data, or give an accurate assessment of plan quality.

[48] Provisions in PPACA that would have (1) required plans to apportion their rebates and bonus payments according to a priority order, and (2) prohibited plans from reducing or eliminating the Part B premium as an additional plan benefit, were overridden by provisions in the reconciliation bill, and thus are not part of the reform law.

[49] Part D premiums are not included in the calculation of a beneficiary's out-of-pocket costs.

[50] Beneficiary cost sharing amounts in 2012 will be 86% of the price of the drug, 79% in 2013, 72% in 2014, 65% in 2015, 58% in 2016, 51% in 2017, 44% in 2018, 37% in 2019, and 25% in 2020.

[51] In a preliminary analysis, CBO estimated that the coverage gap provisions in the PPACA and the Reconciliation Act combined would lead to an average increase in premiums for Part D beneficiaries of about 4% in 2011, rising to about 9% in 2019—an increase of 1% in 2011 and 6% in 2019 from PPACA alone. The increase in premiums is attributed to the increased value of the drug benefit (premiums represent a percentage of total benefit spending). See "Comparison of Projected Medicare Part D Premiums Under Current Law and Under Reconciliation Legislation Combined with H.R. 3590 as Passed by the Senate," March 19, 2010, http://www.cbo.gov/ftpdocs/113xx/doc11355/Comparison.pdf.

[52] In its March 11, 2010, analysis of Section 3301 under H.R. 3590 prior to changes made by the Reconciliation Act, CBO scored the coverage gap discount program alone at a cost of $17.7 billion over 10 years. That projected cost increase was, in part, based on the expectation that under the provision a larger number of enrollees would reach the catastrophic phase when Medicare bears most of the costs, and on the possibility that enrollees who switch from generic to brand-name drugs to take advantage of discounts during the coverage gap may stay on the more expensive brand-name drugs during the catastrophic period.

[53] The effect of the productivity adjustment for home health service is included in the estimate for Sec. 3131.

[54] Name changed from Independent Medicare Advisory Board by Sec. 10320.

[55] The projected Medicare growth rate per beneficiary is to be calculated as a projected five-year average of the growth in Medicare spending. Projections are to assume a zero update in payments for physicians. The projection will also be required to take into account any delivery system reforms or payment changes that have not yet been implemented.

[56] If such a joint resolution were vetoed, it would require a two-third's vote of each chamber to override and enact the measure.

[57] Subtitle F on health care quality improvements is discussed in CRS Report R40943, *Public Health, Workforce, Quality, and Related Provisions in the Patient Protection and Affordable Care Act (P.L. 111-148)*, coordinated by C. Stephen Redhead and Erin D. Williams.

[58] All other provisions in Title IV are addressed in CRS Report R40943, *Public Health, Workforce, Quality, and Related Provisions in the Patient Protection and Affordable Care Act (P.L. 111-148)*, coordinated by C. Stephen Redhead and Erin D. Williams.

[59] An adopted amendment could affect the implementation of several provisions in the PPACA, including sections 4103, 4104, and 4105 (discussed in this report). On December 2, 2009, the Senate adopted S.Amdt. 2808, introduced by Senator Vitter, which would provide that "for the purposes of this Act, and for the purposes of any other provisions of law, the current recommendations of the Unite States Preventive Services Task Force regarding breast cancer screening, mammography, and prevention shall be considered the most current other than those issued in or around November 2009." Previously, the panel had recommended routine screening for women beginning at age 40; in November 2009, it recommended that routine screening begin at age 50. The USPSTF and the relationship between its recommendations and coverage decisions is discussed further in CRS Report R40978, *Medicare Coverage of Clinical Preventive Services*, by Sarah A. Lister and Kirsten J. Colello.

[60] See the U.S. Preventive Services Task Force, http://www.ahrq.gov/clinic/uspstfix.htm.

[61] All other Title V provisions are discussed in CRS Report R40943, *Public Health, Workforce, Quality, and Related Provisions in the Patient Protection and Affordable Care Act (P.L. 111-148)*, coordinated by C. Stephen Redhead and Erin D. Williams.

[62] The preventive services as defined by the PHSA include prenatal and perinatal services; appropriate cancer screening; well-child services; immunizations against vaccine-preventable diseases; screenings for elevated blood lead levels, communicable diseases, and cholesterol; pediatric eye, ear, and dental screenings to determine the need for vision and hearing correction and dental care; voluntary family planning services; preventive dental services.

[63] Subtitle B on nursing home transparency and Subtitle C on background checks are discussed in CRS Report R40943, *Public Health, Workforce, Quality, and Related Provisions in the Patient Protection and Affordable Care Act (P.L. 111-148)*, coordinated by C. Stephen Redhead and Erin D. Williams.

[64] 31 U.S.C. §§ 3729-3733.

[65] 42 U.S.C. § 1320a-7a.

[66] See discussion under the section "Health Care Fraud" for a description of the federal anti-kickback statute.

[67] Provisions in Subtitle F regarding Medicaid program integrity are discussed in CRS Report R41210, *Medicaid and the State Children's Health Insurance Program (CHIP) Provisions in PPACA*, coordinated by Julie Stone.

[68] 18 U.S.C. § 24.

[69] For example, under 18 U.S.C. §1345, the Attorney General may seek injunctive relief and freeze assets for persons committing or about to commit a "federal health care offense."

[70] The March 20, 2010, CBO score does not include changes made by the Manager's amendment to the Reconciliation Act. The prior Section 1303 was deleted and 1304 (as scored by CBO) was renumbered as 1303 in the Reconciliation Act as enacted.

[71] As defined in the Internal Revenue Code (IRC) Sec. 401(a), 403(a), 403(b), 408, 408A, or 457(b).

[72] Modified adjusted gross income is defined as adjusted gross income increased by the excess of foreign earned income (defined in IRC Sec. 911(a)(1)) over the amount of any deductions or exclusions disallowed under IRC Sec. 911(d)(6) when determining foreign earned income.

[73] Corporations may elect S-corporation status if they meet a number of Internal Revenue Code requirements. Among other things, they cannot have more than 100 shareholders or more than one class of stock. S-corporations are tax-reporting rather than tax-paying entities, in contrast to C-corporations, which are subject to the corporate income tax.

[74] For ease of reference to related provision titles in Appendix A, the section numbers of PPACA Title X or Reconciliation Act provisions that modify a PPACA (Title I through IX) provision are included in each line item associated with that PPACA provision, even though that particular implementation date may not be specifically affected by the Title X or Reconciliation Act changes.

In: Medicare and the Patient Protection and Affordable Care Act ISBN: 978-1-61122-897-7
Editor: Paul L. Schmidt

Chapter 2

Medicare Primer*

Patricia A. Davis

Summary

Medicare is a federal insurance program that pays for covered health care services of qualified beneficiaries. It was established in 1965 under Title XVIII of the Social Security Act as a federal entitlement program to provide health insurance to individuals 65 and older, and has been expanded over the years to include permanently disabled individuals under 65. Medicare, which consists of four parts (A-D), covers hospitalizations, physician services, prescription drugs, skilled nursing facility care, home health visits, and hospice care, among other services.

Generally, individuals are eligible for Medicare if they or their spouse worked for at least 40 quarters in Medicare-covered employment, are 65 years old, and are a citizen or permanent resident of the United States. Individuals may also qualify for coverage if they are a younger person with a permanent disability, have End-Stage Renal disease (permanent kidney failure requiring dialysis or transplant), or have amyotrophic lateral sclerosis (ALS, Lou Gehrig's disease).

In FY2010, the program will cover an estimated 47 million persons (39 million aged and 8 million disabled) at an estimated total cost of about $521 billion, accounting for approximately 3.6% of GDP. Medicare is an entitlement program, which means that it is required to pay for services provided to eligible persons so long as specific criteria are met.

Since 1965, the Medicare program has undergone considerable changes. Most recently, the Patient Protection and Affordable Care Act (PPACA, P.L. 111-148) and the Health Care and Education Reconciliation Act of 2010 (HCERA, P.L. 111-152), signed into law on March 23, 2010, and March 30, 2010, respectively, made numerous changes to the Medicare

* This is an edited, reformatted and augmented version of Congressional Research Service publication, Report R40425, dated July 1, 2010.

program that modify provider reimbursements, provide incentives to increase the quality and efficiency of care, and enhance certain Medicare benefits.

Having passed health reform legislation in March 2010, the remaining months of the 111th Congress may be partly spent working on addressing Medicare physician payment issues and on identifying and making any necessary technical fixes to the March legislation. Over the long term, Congress' focus will include monitoring the implementation and effects of payment and program changes made by the new health care reform laws.

This report provides an overview of Medicare and will be updated to reflect any legislative changes.

Introduction

Medicare is a federal insurance program that pays for covered health care services of qualified beneficiaries. It was established in 1965 under Title XVIII of the Social Security Act as a federal entitlement program to provide health insurance to individuals 65 and older, and has been expanded over the years to include permanently disabled individuals under 65. Medicare consists of four distinct parts:

- Part A (Hospital Insurance, or HI) covers inpatient hospital services, skilled nursing care, and home health and hospice care. The HI trust fund is mainly funded by a dedicated payroll tax of 2.9% of earnings, shared equally between employers and workers.
- Part B (Supplementary Medical Insurance, or SMI) covers physician services, outpatient services, and some home health and preventive services. The SMI trust fund is funded through beneficiary premiums (set at 25% of estimated program costs for the aged) and general revenues (the remaining amount, approximately 75%).
- Part C (Medicare Advantage, or MA) is a private plan option for beneficiaries that covers all Part A and B services, except hospice. Individuals choosing to enroll in Part C must also enroll in Part B. Part C is funded through the HI and SMI trust funds.
- Part D covers prescription drug benefits. Funding is included in the SMI trust fund and is financed through beneficiary premiums (about 25.5%) and general revenues (about 74.5%).

Medicare serves approximately one in seven Americans and virtually all of the population aged 65 and over. In 2010, the program will cover an estimated 47 million persons (39 million aged and 8 million disabled). The Congressional Budget Office (CBO) estimates that total Medicare spending in 2010 will be about $521 billion, accounting for approximately 3.6% of GDP. CBO also estimates that federal Medicare spending (after deduction of beneficiary premiums and other offsetting receipts) will be about $444 billion in 2010, accounting for over 15% of total federal spending. Medicare is an entitlement program, which means that it is required to pay for all covered services provided to eligible persons, so long as specific criteria are met. Spending under the program (except for a portion of administrative costs) is considered mandatory spending (not discretionary spending, which is subject to the appropriations process).

Having passed health reform legislation in March 2010, the remaining months of the 111th Congress may be partly spent working on addressing Medicare physician payment issues and on identifying and making any necessary technical fixes to the March legislation. The Committees of jurisdiction for the entitlement (or benefits) portion of Medicare are the Senate Committee on Finance, the House Committee on Ways and Means, and the House Committee on Energy and Commerce. The House and Senate Committees on Appropriations have jurisdiction over the discretionary spending used to administer and oversee the program.

Medicare History

Medicare was enacted in 1965 (P.L. 89-97) in response to the concern that only about half of the nation's seniors had health insurance, and most of those had coverage only for inpatient hospital costs. The new program, which became effective July 1, 1966, included Part A coverage for hospital and post-hospital services and Part B coverage for doctors and other medical services. As is the case for the Social Security program, Part A is financed by payroll taxes levied on current workers and their employers; persons must pay into the system for 40 calendar quarters to become entitled to premium-free benefits. Medicare Part B is voluntary, with a monthly premium required of beneficiaries who choose to enroll. Payments to health care providers under both Part A and Part B were originally based on the most common form of payment at the time, namely "reasonable costs" for hospital and other institutional services or "usual, customary and reasonable charges" (UCR)[1] for physicians and other medical services.

Medicare is considered a social insurance program and is the second largest such federal program, after Social Security. The 1965 law also established Medicaid, the federal/state health insurance program for the poor; this was an expansion of previous welfare-based assistance programs. Some low-income individuals qualify for both Medicare and Medicaid.

In the ensuing 45 years, Medicare has undergone considerable changes. P.L. 92-603, enacted in 1972, expanded program coverage to certain individuals under 65 (the disabled and persons with end-stage renal disease (ESRD)),[2] and introduced managed care into Medicare. This law also began to place limitations on the definitions of reasonable costs and charges in order to gain some control over program spending which, even initially, exceeded original projections.

During the 1980s and 1990s, a number of laws were enacted that included provisions designed to further stem the rapid increase in program spending through modifications to the way payments to providers were determined, and to postpone the bankruptcy of the Medicare Part A trust fund. This was typically achieved through tightening rules governing payments to providers of services and limiting the annual updates in such payments. The program moved from payments based on reasonable costs and reasonable charges to payment systems under which a predetermined payment amount was established for a specified unit of service. At the same time, beneficiaries were given expanded options to obtain covered services through private managed care arrangements, typically health maintenance organizations (HMOs).

Most Medicare payment provisions were incorporated into larger budget reconciliation bills designed to control overall federal spending.

This effort culminated in the enactment of the Balanced Budget Act of 1997 (BBA 97, P.L. 105- 33). This law slowed the rate of growth in payments to providers and established new payment systems for certain categories of providers. It also established the Medicare+Choice program, which expanded private plan options for beneficiaries and changed the way most of these plans were paid. BBA 97 further expanded preventive services covered by the program.

Subsequently, Congress became concerned that the BBA 97 cuts in payments to providers were somewhat larger than originally anticipated. Therefore, legislation was enacted in both 1999 (Balanced Budget Refinement Act of 1999, BBRA, P.L. 106-113) and 2000 (Medicare, Medicaid, and SCHIP Benefits Improvement and Protection Act of 2000, BIPA, P.L. 106-554) to mitigate the impact of BBA 97 on providers.

In 2003, Congress enacted the Medicare Prescription Drug, Improvement, and Modernization Act of 2003 (MMA, P.L. 108-173),[3] which included a major benefit expansion and placed increasing emphasis on the private sector to deliver and manage benefits. The MMA included provisions that (1) created a new voluntary outpatient prescription drug benefit to be administered by private entities; (2) replaced the Medicare+Choice program with the Medicare Advantage (MA) program and raised payments to plans in order to increase their availability for beneficiaries; (3) introduced the concept of income testing into Medicare, with higher-income persons paying larger Part B premiums beginning in 2007; (4) modified some provider payment rules; (5) expanded covered preventive services; and (6) created a specific process for overall program review if general revenue spending exceeded a specified threshold.

During the 109th Congress, two laws were enacted that incorporated minor modifications to Medicare's payment rules. These were the Deficit Reduction Act of 2005 (DRA, P.L. 109-171) and the Tax Relief and Health Care Act of 2006 (TRHCA, P.L. 109-432). In the 110th Congress, additional changes were incorporated in the Medicare, Medicaid, and SCHIP Extension Act of 2007 (MMSEA, P.L. 1 10-173)[4] and the Medicare Improvements for Patients and Providers Act of 2008 (MIPPA, P.L. 110-275).[5]

In the 111th Congress, comprehensive health reform legislation was enacted that, among other things, made statutory changes to the Medicare program. The Patient Protection and Affordable Care Act (PPACA; P.L. 111-148), enacted on March 23, 2010, included numerous provisions affecting Medicare payments, payment rules, covered benefits, and the delivery of care. The Health Care and Education Affordability Reconciliation Act of 2010 (the Reconciliation Act, or HCERA; P.L. 111-152), enacted on March 30, 2010, made changes to a number of Medicare- related provisions in PPACA and added several new provisions.[6] Included in these new laws are provisions that (1) constrain Medicare's annual payment increases for certain providers; (2) change payment rates in the Medicare Advantage program so that they more closely resemble those in fee-for-service; (3) reduce payments to hospitals that serve a large number of low-income patients; (4) create an Independent Payment Advisory Board that will make recommendations to adjust Medicare payment rates; (5) phase out the Part D prescription drug benefit "doughnut hole"; and (6) provide incentives to increase the quality and efficiency of care, such as creating value-based purchasing programs for certain types of providers, allowing accountable care organizations (ACOs) that meet certain quality and efficiency standards to share in the savings,[7] creating a voluntary pilot program that bundles payments for physician, hospital, and post-acute care services, and adjusting payments to hospitals for readmissions related to certain potentially preventable conditions.

Eligibility and Enrollment

Most persons aged 65 or older are automatically entitled to premium-free Part A because they or their spouse paid Medicare payroll taxes for at least 40 quarters (10 years) on earnings covered by either the Social Security or the Railroad Retirement systems. Persons under age 65 who receive cash disability benefits from Social Security or the Railroad Retirement systems for at least 24 months are also entitled to Part A. (Since there is a five-month waiting period for cash payments, the Medicare waiting period is effectively 29 months.)[8] The 24-month waiting period is waived for persons with amyotrophic lateral sclerosis (ALS, "Lou Gehrig's disease"). Individuals of any age with ESRD who receive dialysis on a regular basis or a kidney transplant are eligible for Medicare. Medicare coverage for individuals with ESRD usually starts the first day of the fourth month of dialysis treatments.

Persons over age 65 who are not automatically entitled to Part A may obtain coverage by paying a monthly premium ($461 in 2010) or, for persons with at least 30 quarters of covered employment, a reduced monthly premium ($254 in 2010). In addition, disabled persons who lose their cash benefits solely because of higher earnings, and subsequently lose their extended Medicare coverage, may continue their Medicare enrollment by paying a premium, subject to limitations.

Generally, enrollment in Medicare Part B is voluntary. All persons entitled to Part A (and persons over 65 not entitled to premium-free Part A) may enroll in Part B by paying a monthly premium. For established Part B enrollees, the 2010 monthly premium remains at $96.40.[9] Beginning in 2007, some higher-income individuals started to pay higher premiums. (See the "Part B" section, below.) While enrollment in Part B is voluntary for most individuals, those who voluntarily enroll in Part A must also enroll in Part B. Additionally, ESRD beneficiaries and Medicare Advantage enrollees (discussed below) must also enroll in Part B.

Together, Parts A and B of Medicare comprise "original Medicare," which covers benefits on a fee-for-service (FFS) basis. Beneficiaries have another option for coverage through private plans, called the Medicare Advantage (MA or Part C) program. When beneficiaries first become eligible for Medicare, they may chose either original Medicare or they may enroll in a private MA plan. Each fall, there is an annual open enrollment period during which time Medicare beneficiaries may choose a different MA plan, or leave or join the MA program. [10] In 2010, the annual open enrollment period will be from November 15 to December 31 for plan choices effective in 2011. Starting in 2011, the annual open enrollment period will be from October 15 to December 7 for plan choices starting the following January.

Finally, each individual enrolled in either Part A or Part B is also entitled to obtain qualified prescription drug coverage through enrollment in a Part D prescription drug plan. Similar to Part B, enrollment in Part D is voluntary and the beneficiary pays a monthly premium. Beginning in 2011, some higher-income enrollees will pay higher premiums, similar to enrollees in Part B. Generally, beneficiaries enrolled in an MA plan providing qualified prescription drug coverage (MA-PD plan) must obtain their prescription drug coverage through that plan.[11]

In general, individuals who do not enroll in Part B or Part D during an initial enrollment period (when they first become eligible for Medicare) must pay a permanent penalty of increased monthly premiums if they choose to enroll at a later date. Individuals who do not enroll in Part B during their initial enrollment period may enroll only during the annual open enrollment period, which occurs from January 1–March 31 each year. Coverage begins the following July 1. However, the law waives the Part B late enrollment penalty for current workers who have primary coverage through their own or a spouse's employer-sponsored plan. These individuals have a special enrollment period once their employment ends; as long as they enroll in Part B during this time, they will not be subject to penalty.

Individuals who do not enroll in Part D during their initial enrollment period may enroll during the annual open enrollment period, which corresponds with the Part C annual enrollment period—in 2010, from November 15 to December 31, and in 2011 and future years, from October 15 to December 7, with coverage effective the following January. Individuals are not subject to the Part D penalty if they have maintained "creditable" drug coverage through another source, such as retiree health coverage offered by a former employer or union. However, once employees retire or have no access to "creditable" Part D coverage, a penalty will apply unless they sign up for coverage during a special enrollment period. Finally, for persons who qualify for the low-income subsidy for Part D, the delayed-enrollment penalty does not apply.

Benefits and Payments

Medicare Parts A, B, and D each cover different services, with Part C providing a private plan alternative for Medicare services, except hospice. The Parts A-D covered services are described below, along with a description of Medicare's payments.

Part A

Part A provides coverage for inpatient hospital services, post-hospital skilled nursing facility (SNF) services, post-hospital home health services, and hospice care, subject to certain conditions and limitations. Approximately 20% of Part A enrollees use Part A services during a year.

Inpatient Hospital Services

Medicare inpatient hospital services include (1) bed and board; (2) nursing services; (3) use of hospital facilities; (4) drugs, biologics, supplies, appliances, and equipment; and (5) diagnostic and therapeutic items and services. (Physicians' services provided during an inpatient stay are paid under the physician fee schedule and discussed below in the "Physicians and Non-physician Practitioner Services" section.) Coverage for inpatient services is linked to an individual's benefit period or "spell of illness" (defined as beginning on the day a patient enters a hospital and ending when he or she has not been in a hospital or

SNF for 60 days). An individual admitted to a hospital more than 60 days after the last discharge from a hospital or SNF begins a new benefit period. Coverage in each benefit period is subject to the following conditions:

- Days 1-60. Beneficiary pays a deductible ($1,100 in 2010).
- Days 6 1-90. Beneficiary pays a daily coinsurance charge ($275 in 2010).
- Days 9 1-150. After 90 days, the beneficiary may draw on one or more of 60 lifetime reserve days, provided they have not been previously used. (Each of the 60 lifetime reserve days can be used only once during an individual's lifetime.) For lifetime reserve days, the beneficiary pays a daily coinsurance charge ($550 in 2010); otherwise the beneficiary pays all costs.
- Days 151 and over. Beneficiary pays for all costs for these days.

Inpatient mental health care in a psychiatric facility is limited to 190 days during a patient's lifetime. Cost sharing is structured similarly to that for stays in a general hospital (above).

Medicare makes payments to most acute care hospitals under the inpatient prospective payment (IPPS) system, using a prospectively determined amount for each discharge. Medicare's payments to hospitals is the product of two components: (1) a discharge payment amount adjusted by a wage index for the area where the hospital is located or where it has been reclassified, and (2) the weight associated with the Medicare severity-diagnosis related group (MS-DRG) to which the patient is assigned. This weight reflects the relative costliness of the average patient in that MS-DRG, which is revised annually, generally effective October 1 of each year.

Additional payments are made to hospitals for cases with extraordinary costs (outliers), indirect costs incurred by teaching hospitals for graduate medical education, and disproportionate share hospital (DSH) payments to those hospitals serving a certain volume of low-income patients. Additional payments may also be made for qualified new technologies that have been approved for special add-on payments. Prospective payments are also made for inpatient capital costs.

Medicare also makes payments outside the IPPS system for direct costs associated with graduate medical education (GME) for hospital residents, subject to certain limits. In addition, Medicare reimburses hospitals for 70% of the allowable costs associated with beneficiaries' unpaid deductible and copayment amounts as well as for the costs for certain other services.

Additional payments or special treatment may apply for hospitals meeting one of the following designations: (1) sole community hospitals (SCHs), (2) Medicare dependent hospitals, and (3) rural referral centers. Certain hospitals or distinct hospital units are exempt from IPPS and paid on an alternative basis,[12] including (1) inpatient rehabilitation facilities, (2) long-term care hospitals, (3) psychiatric facilities including hospitals and distinct part units, (4) children's hospitals and cancer hospitals, and (5) critical access hospitals.

Skilled Nursing Facility (SNF) Services

Medicare covers up to 100 days of post-hospital care for persons needing skilled nursing or rehabilitation services on a daily basis. The SNF stay must be preceded by a hospital stay of at least three days, and the transfer to the SNF must occur within 30 days of the hospital discharge. There is no beneficiary cost-sharing for the first 20 days. Days 21-100 are subject to daily coinsurance charges ($137.50 in 2010). The 100-day limit begins again with a new spell of illness.

SNF services are paid under a prospective payment system (PPS), which is based on a per diem urban or rural base payment rate, adjusted for case mix (average severity of illness) and area wages. The per diem rate generally covers all services, including room and board, provided to the patient that day. The case-mix adjustment is made using the resource utilization groups (RUGs) system, which uses patient assessments to assign a beneficiary to one of 53 categories that reflect the beneficiary's expected use of services. Patient assessments are done at various times during a patient's stay and the RUG category a beneficiary is placed in can change with changes in the beneficiary's condition. Extra payments are not made for extraordinarily costly cases ("outliers").

Home Health Services

Medicare covers visits by participating home health agencies for beneficiaries who (1) are confined to home, (2) need skilled nursing care on an intermittent basis, or (3) need physical or occupational therapy or speech language therapy. After establishing such eligibility, the continuing need for occupational therapy services may extend the eligibility period. Covered services include part-time or intermittent nursing care, physical or occupational therapy or speech language pathology services, medical social services, home health aide services, and medical supplies and durable medical equipment. The services must be provided under a plan of care established by a physician, and the plan must be reviewed by the physician at least every 60 days.

Home health services are covered under both Medicare Parts A and B. Part A covers up to 100 visits following a stay in a hospital or SNF. Part A also covers all home health services for persons not enrolled in Part B. All other home health services are covered under Part B. There is no beneficiary cost-sharing for home health services (though some other Part B services provided in connection with the visit, such as durable medical equipment, are subject to cost-sharing charges).

Home health services are paid under a home health PPS, based on 60-day episodes of care; a patient may have an unlimited number of episodes. Under the PPS, a nationwide base payment amount is adjusted by differences in wages (using the hospital wage index). This amount is then adjusted for case mix using the applicable Home Health Resource Group (HHRG) to which the beneficiary has been assigned. The HHRG applicable to a beneficiary is determined following an assessment of the patient's condition and care needs using the Outcome and Assessment Information Set (OASIS); there are 153 HHRGs. Further payment adjustments may be made for outlier visits (for extremely costly patients), a significant change in a beneficiary's condition, a partial episode which occurs because a beneficiary transfers from one agency to another, or a low utilization adjustment for beneficiaries receiving four or fewer visits.

Hospice Care

The Medicare hospice benefit covers services designed to provide palliative care and management of a terminal illness; the benefit includes drugs and medical and support services. These services are provided to Medicare beneficiaries with a life expectancy of six months or less for two 90-day periods, followed by an unlimited number of 60-day periods.

The individual's attending physician and the hospice physician must certify the need for the first benefit period, but only the hospice physician needs to recertify for subsequent periods. Starting January 1, 2011, a hospice physician or nurse practitioner must have a face-to-face encounter with the individual to determine continued eligibility prior to the 180th day recertification, and for each subsequent recertification. Hospice care is provided in lieu of most other Medicare services related to the curative treatment of the terminal illness. Beneficiaries electing hospice care from a hospice program may receive curative services for illnesses or injuries unrelated to their terminal illness and they may disenroll from the hospice at any time. Nominal cost-sharing is required for drugs and respite care.

Payment for hospice care is based on one of four prospectively determined rates (which correspond to four different levels of care) for each day a beneficiary is under the care of the hospice. The four rate categories are routine home care, continuous home care, inpatient respite care, and general inpatient care. Payment rates are adjusted to reflect differences in area wage levels, using the hospital wage index.[13] Payments to a hospice are subject to an aggregate cap that limits the average per beneficiary cost to a cap that is adjusted annually by changes to the medical care expenditure category of the Consumer Price Index for all urban consumers (CPI-U).

Part A Services for End-Stage Renal Disease (ESRD)

Individuals with ESRD (i.e., kidney disease) are eligible for all services covered under Parts A and B. Kidney transplantation services, to the extent they are inpatient hospital services, are subject to the inpatient hospital PPS. However, kidney acquisition costs are paid on a reasonable cost basis. (See "Part B Services for End-Stage Renal Disease" for an explanation of dialysis benefits and payments, as well as other Part B ESRD services.)

Part B

Medicare Part B covers physicians' services, outpatient hospital services, durable medical equipment, and other medical services. Initially, over 98% of the eligible population voluntarily enrolled in Part B, but in recent years, the percentage has fallen to about 92%.[14] Over 80% of Part B enrollees use Part B services during a year. The program generally pays 80% of the approved amount (most commonly, a fee schedule or other predetermined amount) for covered services in excess of the annual deductible ($155 in 2010). The beneficiary is liable for the remaining 20%.

Most providers and practitioners are subject to limits on amounts they can bill beneficiaries for covered services. For example, physicians and some other practitioners may choose whether or not to accept "assignment" on a claim. When a physician accepts assignment, the physician can only bill the beneficiary the 20% coinsurance plus any unmet deductible. When a physician agrees to accept assignment on all Medicare claims in a given year, the physician is referred to as a "participating physician." Physicians who do not agree to accept assignment on all Medicare claims in a given year are referred to as nonparticipating physicians. Nonparticipating physicians may or may not accept assignment for a given service. If they do not, they may charge beneficiaries more than the fee schedule amount on nonassigned claims; however, these "balance billing" charges are subject to certain limits.

Additionally, other providers may choose not to accept any Medicare payment and enter into a private contracts with their patients.

For some providers, such as nurse practitioners and physician assistants, assignment is mandatory; these providers can only bill the beneficiary the 20% coinsurance and any unmet deductible. For other Part B services, such as durable medical equipment, assignment is optional; for these services, applicable providers may bill beneficiaries for amounts above Medicare's recognized payment level and may do so without limit.

Physicians and Non-physician Practitioner Services

Medicare Part B covers medically necessary doctors' services, outpatient care, home health services, some preventive care, and some other medical services. Certain limitations apply for services provided by chiropractors and podiatrists. Beneficiary cost-sharing is typically 20% of the approved amount, although preventive care services require no coinsurance from the beneficiary and outpatient mental health services are currently in the first of a five-year phase-in that will reduce beneficiary responsibility from 50% to 20% by 2014.[15] Covered non-physician practitioner services include, but are not limited to, those provided by physician assistants, nurse practitioners, certified registered nurse anesthetists, and clinical social workers.

A number of Part B services are paid under the physician fee schedule. These include services of physicians, non-physician practitioners, and therapists. Most services described below as preventive services (except for laboratory tests paid under the laboratory fee schedule) and diagnostic tests are paid under the physician fee schedule. There are over 7,000 service codes under the fee schedule.

The fee schedule assigns relative values to each service code. These relative values reflect physician work (based on time, skill, and intensity involved), practice expenses, and malpractice expenses. The relative values are adjusted for geographic variations in the costs of practicing medicine. These geographically adjusted relative values are converted into a dollar payment amount by a national conversion factor. The conversion factor is updated each year by a formula specified in law. The update percentage is based on the Medicare Economic Index (MEI, which measures changes in the prices of the inputs required to provide physician services) subject to an adjustment to match spending under the cumulative sustainable growth rate (SGR) system, which establishes a target for total expenditures since 1996. If total expenditures exceed the target, the update for a future year is reduced. Application of the SGR formula would have led to negative updates each year since 2002. However, Congress has acted several times to avert reductions, thereby overriding the statutory formula for the 2003-20 10 period. The update to the conversion factor for 2009 was 1.1% above that for 2008, and the update for January through May 2010 has been 0%. The update to the conversion factor for June through November 2010 is 2.2%. Beginning December 2010, a substantial reduction will be required absent additional action by Congress.[16]

In addition to the fee schedule reimbursements, physicians who report on selected quality measures for services for which quality measures are established will receive bonus payments for those services provided from July 2007 to December 2010. The bonus payments were 1.5% during the second half of 2007 and for 2008, and 2.0% for 2009 and 2010. The bonuses will diminish to 1% in 2011 and to 0.5% in 2012, 2013, and 2014 for those who successfully report the measures. Subsequently, those providers who fail to successfully report the measures will be subject to a 1.5% penalty in 2015 and a 2% penalty in 2016 and future years.

Additional bonus payments will be made for 2009-2013 for Medicare professionals providing covered services who are successful electronic prescribers and in 2011-2014 for those who meet the requirements of a Maintenance of Certification Program (MOCP).[17]

Therapy Services

Medicare therapy services include physical therapy, occupational therapy, and speech language pathology services. The program establishes annual limits (therapy caps) on covered services. The first is a $1,860 per beneficiary annual cap in 2010 for all outpatient physical therapy services and speech language pathology services. The second is a $1,860 per beneficiary annual cap in 2010 for all outpatient occupational therapy services. The limits, which are updated annually, apply to services provided by independent therapists as well as to those provided by comprehensive outpatient rehabilitation facilities (CORFs) and other rehabilitation agencies. The Secretary is required to implement an exceptions process, effective from 2006 through 2010, for services meeting specified criteria for medically necessary services. The limits do not apply to outpatient services provided by hospitals.

Preventive Services

The original Medicare statutes prohibited payment for covered items and services that are "not reasonable and necessary for the diagnosis or treatment of illness or injury or to improve the functioning of a malformed body member," which effectively excluded preventive and screening services. In recent years, Congress has added and expanded Medicare coverage for a number of such services through legislation, including MMA, MIPPA, and PPACA. Coverage for preventive and screening services currently includes the following: (1) a "welcome to Medicare" physical exam during the first year of enrollment in Part B and an annual visit and prevention plan thereafter; (2) flu vaccine (annual), pneumococcal vaccine (usually needed only once in a lifetime), and hepatitis B vaccine (for persons at high risk); (3) annual screening mammograms for asymptomatic women 40 and over; (4) PAP smears and pelvic exams; (5) several types of colorectal cancer screening tests; (6) prostate cancer screening; (7) certain screening tests for heart disease; (8) bone mass measurement; (9) diabetes screening and self-management training; (10) glaucoma tests; (11) medical nutrition therapy (MNT) services; (12) ultrasound screening for abdominal aortic aneurysms; and (13) HIV screening for persons at high risk; and (14) others determined by the Secretary of Health and Human Services, under certain conditions. These services are covered under the Medicare Part B fee schedule. Deductibles and cost-sharing are waived.

Clinical Lab and other Diagnostic Tests

Part B covers clinical laboratory tests. Neither copayment nor deductible applies to services paid under the Medicare clinical laboratory fee schedule. There is no coinsurance for clinical laboratory services. Clinical lab services are paid on the basis of area-wide fee schedules. There is a ceiling on payment amounts equal to 74% of the median of all fee schedules for the test. In general, annual increases in clinical lab fees are based on the percentage change in the CPI-U. However, Congress has modified the update in recent years, by (1) freezing the fee schedule amounts through 2008 and (2) reducing the update that would otherwise apply by 0.5 percentage points each year, for 2009-2013.

Part B also covers diagnostic x-ray tests and other diagnostic tests, as well as x-ray, radium, and radioisotope therapy. Generally, these services are paid for under the physician fee schedule.

Durable Medical Equipment, Prosthetics, Orthotics and Supplies (DMEPOS)

Medicare covers a wide variety of equipment and devices under the heading of durable medical equipment (DME), and prosthetics, orthotics (PO) if they are medically necessary and are prescribed by a physician. DME is defined as equipment that (1) can withstand repeated use, (2) is used primarily to serve a medical purpose, (3) is not generally useful in the absence of an illness or injury, and (4) is appropriate for use in the home. DME includes such items as hospital beds, wheelchairs, blood glucose monitors, and oxygen and oxygen equipment. It also includes related supplies, such as drugs and biologics that are necessary for the effective use of the product. PO is defined as items that replace all or part of a body organ, such as colostomy bags and pacemakers, as well as leg, arm, back, and neck braces and artificial legs, arms, and eyes. Medicare also covers some items or supplies (S), such as disposable surgical dressings that do not meet the definitions of DME or PO.

Except in competitive bidding areas (described below), Medicare pays for most DMEPOS based on fee schedules. Medicare pays 80% of the lower of the supplier's charge for the item or the fee schedule amount. The beneficiary is responsible for the remaining 20%. In general, fee schedule amounts are updated each year by a measure of price inflation, but Congress has specified a reduction or elimination in updates in recent years.

Numerous studies and investigations have shown that Medicare payments for certain items of DME and PO are higher than those made by other health insurers and some retail outlets.[18] Such overpayments may be due partly to the fee schedule mechanism of payment. MMA required the Secretary to establish a Competitive Acquisition Program for certain DMEPOS in specified areas. Instead of paying for medical equipment based on a fee schedule established by law, payment for items would be determined based on the supplier bids. The bids would determine how much suppliers were "willing to accept" to furnish different items. MIPPA delayed the program and required the first round of the program to be re-bid, in addition to other changes. The re-bid took place in 2009 and the program is estimated to start in January 2011.[19]

Part B Drugs and Biologics[20]

Certain specified outpatient prescription drugs and biologics are covered under Medicare Part B. (However, most outpatient prescription drugs are covered under Part D, discussed below.) Covered Part B drugs and biologics include drugs furnished incident to physicians' services, immunosuppressive drugs following a Medicare-covered organ transplant, erythropoietin for treatment of anemia for persons with ESRD, oral anti-cancer drugs (provided they have the same active ingredients and are used for the same indications as chemotherapy drugs which would be covered if furnished incident to physicians services), and drugs needed for the effective use of DME. Generally, Medicare's payment for Part B covered drugs equals 106% of the average sales price.

Hospital Outpatient Department Services

Hospitals provide two distinct types of services to outpatients: services that are diagnostic in nature, and other services that aid the physician in the treatment of the patient. A hospital outpatient is a person who has not been admitted by the hospital as an inpatient but is registered on the hospital records as an outpatient. Generally, payments under the hospital outpatient prospective payment system (OPPS) cover the operating and capital-related costs that are directly related and integral to performing a procedure or furnishing a service on an outpatient basis. These payments cover services such as the use of an operating suite, treatment, procedure or recovery room; use of an observations bed as well as anesthesia; certain drugs or pharmaceuticals; incidental services; and other necessary or implantable supplies or services. Payments for services such as those provided by physicians and other professionals as well as therapy and clinical diagnostic laboratory services, among others, are separate.

Under the OPPS, the unit of payment for acute care hospitals is the individual service or procedure as assigned to an ambulatory payment classification (APC). To the extent possible, integral services and items (excluding physician services paid under the physician fee schedule) are bundled within each APC. Specified new technologies are assigned to "new technology APCs" until clinical and cost data are available to permit assignment into a "clinical APC."

Medicare's hospital outpatient payment is calculated by multiplying the relative weight associated with an APC by a conversion factor. For most APCs, 60% of the conversion factor is geographically adjusted by the wage index used for the inpatient prospective payment system. Except for new technology APCs, each APC has a relative weight that is based on the median cost of services in that APC. The OPPS also includes pass-through payments for new technologies (specific drugs, biologicals, and devices) and payments for outliers.[21]

Ambulatory Surgical Center Services

Medicare covers surgical and medical services performed in an ambulatory surgical center (ASC) that are (1) commonly performed on an inpatient basis but may be safely performed in an ASC; (2) not of a type that are commonly performed or that may be safely performed in physicians' offices; (3) limited to procedures requiring a dedicated operating room or suite and generally requiring a post-operative recovery room or short term (not overnight) convalescent room; and (4) not otherwise excluded from Medicare coverage.

Beginning in January 2008, Medicare pays for surgery-related facility services provided in ASCs using a payment system based on the OPPS. (Associated physician fees are paid for separately under the physician fee schedule.) Each of the 3,300 procedures approved for payment in an ASC is classified into an ambulatory payment classification (APC) group on the basis of clinical and cost similarity. The ASC system uses the same payment groups (APCs) as the OPPS, and for most procedures, the same relative weights used in the OPPS also apply. The ASC system uses a conversion factor based on a percentage of the OPPS conversion factor. The percentage of this average dollar figure is set to ensure budget neutrality, so that total payments under the new ASC payment system should equal total payments under the old ASC payment system. A different payment method is used to set ASC payment for new, office-based procedures, separately payable drugs, and device-intensive procedures.[22] This policy also applies to separately payable radiology services. Separately payable drugs in an ASC are paid the same amount as if provided in a hospital outpatient department. Different rules apply for device intensive procedures (where a device that is packaged into an APC accounts for more than half of its total payments). Separate payments are made for corneal tissue acquisition, brachytherapy sources, certain radiology services, many drugs, and certain implantable devices.

Ambulance

Medicare Part B covers ambulance services provided by qualified suppliers, paid for on the basis of a fee schedule. The fee schedule establishes seven categories of ground ambulance services and two categories of air ambulance services. There is a national fee schedule for air ambulance services. For ground ambulance services, payments through 2009 are equal to the greater of the national fee schedule or a blend of 80% national and 20% regional fee schedule amounts. Beginning in 2010, the payments in all areas will be based on the national fee schedule amount.

The payment for a service equals a base rate for the level of service plus payment for mileage, with geographic adjustments made to a portion of the base rate. Additionally, the base rate is increased for air ambulance trips originating in rural areas and mileage payments are increased for all trips originating in rural areas.

Rural Health Clinics and Federally Qualified Health Centers

Medicare covers Part B services in rural health clinics (RHCs) and federally qualified health centers (FQHCs) provided by (1) physicians and specified non-physician practitioners; (2) visiting nurses for homebound patients in home health shortage areas; (3) registered dieticians or nutritional professionals for diabetes training and medical nutrition therapy; and (4) others, as well as otherwise covered drugs.

RHCs and FQHCs are paid based on an "all-inclusive" rate per beneficiary visit subject to a per visit upper limit, adjusted annually for inflation.

Part B Services for End-Stage Renal Disease

Individuals with ESRD are eligible for all Part B Services. Part B also covers their dialysis services, drugs, biologicals (including erythropoiesis stimulating agents (ESAs) for the treatment of ESRD), diagnostic laboratory tests, and other items and services furnished to individuals for the treatment of ESRD.

Dialysis services are offered in three outpatient settings: hospital-based facilities, independent facilities, and the patient's home. There are two methods for payment. Under Method I, facilities are paid a prospectively set amount, known as the composite rate, for each dialysis session. The composite rate is derived from audited cost data and adjusted for the national proportion of patients dialyzing at home versus in a facility, and for area wage differences.

Beneficiaries electing home dialysis may choose to be paid under Method I. Alternatively, a home dialysis beneficiary may choose to not be associated with a facility and may make independent arrangements with a supplier for equipment, supplies, and support services. Payment to these suppliers, known as Method II, is made on the basis of reasonable charges, limited to 100% of the median hospital composite rate, except for patients on continuous cycling peritoneal dialysis, when the limit is 130% of the median hospital composite rate. The composite rate is case-mixed adjusted.

Beginning January 1, 2011, Medicare dialysis payments will be bundled (phased in over four years) using a single payment for Medicare renal dialysis services that includes (1) items and services included in the composite rate as of December 31, 2010; (2) erythropoiesis stimulating agents (ESAs) for the treatment of ESRD; (3) other drugs and biologicals for which payment was made separately (before bundling); and (4) diagnostic laboratory tests and other items and services furnished to individuals for the treatment of ESRD. The new system will be case-mix adjusted based on factors such as patient weight, body mass index, comorbidities, length of time on dialysis, age, race, ethnicity, and other appropriate factors as determined by the Secretary of Health and Human Services.

Part C, Medicare Advantage

Medicare Advantage (MA) is an alternative way for Medicare beneficiaries to receive covered benefits. Under MA, private health plans are paid a per-person amount to provide all Medicare covered benefits (except hospice) to beneficiaries who enroll in their plan. Medicare beneficiaries who are eligible for Part A, enrolled in Part B, and do not have ESRD are eligible to enroll in an MA plan if one is available in their area. Some MA plans may choose the areas they wish to serve (local MA plans), while others agree to serve one or more regions defined by the Secretary (regional MA plans). As of June 2010, all Medicare beneficiaries had access to an MA plan and 25% of beneficiaries enrolled in one. Private plans may use different techniques to influence the medical care used by enrollees. Some plans, such as health maintenance organizations (HMOs), may require enrollees to receive care from a restricted network of medical providers; enrollees may be required to see a primary care physician who will coordinate their care and refer them to specialists as necessary. Other types of private plans, such as private fee-for-service (PFFS) plans, may look more like original Medicare, with fewer restrictions on the providers an enrollee can see and minimal coordination of care.

In general, MA plans offer additional benefits or require smaller co-payments or deductibles than original Medicare. Sometimes beneficiaries pay for these additional benefits through a higher monthly premium, but sometimes they are financed through plan savings. The extent of extra benefits and reduced cost-sharing varies by plan type and geography. However, Medicare Advantage plans are seen by some as an attractive alternative to more expensive supplemental insurance policies found in the private market.

Under an agreement with CMS, a plan agrees to provide all required services covered in return for a capitated monthly payment. The same monthly payment is made regardless of how many or few services a beneficiary actually uses. The plan is at-risk if costs, in the aggregate, exceed program payments; conversely, the plan can retain savings if costs are less than payments. Payments to MA plans are based on a comparison of each plan's estimated cost of providing Medicare covered services (a bid) relative to the maximum amount the federal government will pay for providing those services in the plan's service area (a benchmark). If a plan's bid is less than the benchmark, its payment equals its bid plus a rebate. Currently, the rebate is equal to 75% of the difference (between the benchmark and the bid); starting in 2012, the size of the rebate will be dependent on plan quality. The rebate must be returned to enrollees in the form of either additional benefits, reduced cost-sharing, reduced Part B or Part D premiums, or some combination of these options. If a plan's bid is equal to or above the benchmark, its payment will be the benchmark amount and each enrollee in that plan will pay an additional premium, equal to the amount by which the bid exceeds the benchmark.

The MA benchmarks are determined through statutorily specified formulas that have changed over time. Since BBA 97, formulas have increased the benchmark amounts, in part, to encourage plan participation in all areas of the country. As a result, however, the benchmark amounts (and plan payments) in some areas are higher than the average cost of original FFS Medicare. Most recently, PPACA changed the way benchmarks are to be calculated by tying them closer to (or below) spending in FFS Medicare, and adjusting them based on plan quality. The Congressional Budget Office expects these changes will result in reduced MA enrollment and plan subsidies for extra benefits, though the impact may vary by market.

In 2006, the MA program began to offer MA regional plans. Regional MA plans must agree to serve one or more regions designated by the Secretary. There are 26 MA regions consisting of states or groups of states. Regional plan benchmarks include two components: (1) a statutorily determined amount (comparable to benchmarks described above) and (2) a weighted average of plan bids. Thus, a portion of the benchmark is competitively determined. Similar to local plans, plans with bids below the benchmark are given a rebate, while plans with bids above the benchmark require an additional enrollee premium.

In general, MA eligible individuals may enroll in any MA plan that serves their area. However, some MA plans may restrict their enrollment to beneficiaries who meet additional criteria. For example, employer-sponsored MA plans are generally only available to the retirees of the company sponsoring the plan. In addition, Medicare Special Needs Plans (SNPs) are a type of coordinated care MA plan that exclusively enrolls, or enrolls a disproportionate percentage of, special needs individuals. Special needs individuals are any MA eligible individuals who are either institutionalized as defined by the Secretary, eligible for both Medicare and Medicaid, or have a severe or disabling chronic condition and would benefit from enrollment in a specialized MA plan.

Part D

Part D of Medicare covers outpatient prescription drugs. (As previously discussed, Part B provides limited coverage of some outpatient prescription drugs.) Qualified Part D prescription drug plans are required to offer either "standard coverage" or alternative coverage that has actuarially equivalent benefits. In 2010, "standard coverage" has a $310 deductible and a 25% coinsurance for costs between $310 and $2,830. From this point, there is no coverage until the beneficiary has out-of-pocket costs of $4,550 ($6,440 in total spending); this coverage gap has been labeled the "doughnut hole." Once the beneficiary reaches the catastrophic limit, the program pays all costs except for nominal cost-sharing. In 2010, Medicare is sending tax free, one-time $250 rebate checks to Part D enrollees who reach the doughnut hole. Starting in 2011, the coverage gap will be gradually reduced each year until it is eliminated in 2020.[23] Most plans offer actuarially equivalent benefits rather than the standard package, including alternatives such as reducing or eliminating the deductible, using tiered cost-sharing with lower cost-sharing for generic drugs, or coverage in the doughnut hole.

Part D plan sponsors determine payments for drugs and are expected to negotiate prices. The federal government is prohibited from interfering in the price negotiations between drug manufacturers, pharmacies, and plans (the so-called "non-interference clause").

Part D also provides enhanced coverage for low-income enrolled individuals, such as persons who previously received drug benefits under Medicaid (known as "dual eligibles"—enrollees in both Medicare and Medicaid). Additionally, persons with incomes below 150% of poverty receive assistance for some portion of their premium and cost-sharing charges.

MMA included significant incentives for employers to continue to offer coverage to their retirees by providing a 28% federal subsidy. In 2010, the maximum potential subsidy per covered retiree is $1,677.20 for employers or unions offering drug coverage that is at least actuarially equivalent (called "creditable" coverage), to standard coverage. Employers or unions may select an alternative option (instead of taking the subsidy) with respect to Part D, such as electing to pay a portion of the Part D premiums. They may also elect to provide enhanced coverage, though this has some financial consequences for the employer or union. Alternatively, employers or unions may contract with a PDP or MA-PD to offer the coverage or become a Part D plan sponsor themselves for their retirees.

Administration

At the federal level, Medicare is administered by the Centers for Medicare and Medicaid Services (CMS) within the Department of Health and Human Services (HHS). Medicare statute delegates much of the day-to-day administration of the program to private contractors. Functions such as paying providers (processing reimbursement claims), enrolling providers and suppliers in the Medicare program, educating providers about Medicare billing requirements, and processing appeals are performed by Medicare Administrative Contractors (MACs), Fiscal Intermediaries (FIs), and carriers. Generally, MACs perform these functions for Parts A and B providers, FIs for Part A providers, and carriers for Part B providers. In 2003, MMA required the Secretary to implement FFS contracting reform and replace FIs and carriers with MACs by 2011. CMS has contracted with 15 A/B MACs to process Part A and B claims and four DME MACs to process DME supplier claims. Unlike the prior claims administration contracts, MAC contracts are competitively selected and re-competed every five years.

Under authority provided in the Health Insurance Portability and Accountability Act of 1996 (HIPAA, P.L. 104-191), Medicare contracts with private organizations to protect the Medicare trust funds from making improper payments and fraud and abuse.[24] In addition, to reduce improper Medicare payments, CMS contracts with other private entities, called Recovery Audit Contractors (RACs). In MMA, Congress authorized a three-year demonstration to test RACs, but in 2006, Congress required the program to be expanded nationwide by 2010 when it passed TRHCA. PPACA required the Secretary to expand RACs to Medicare Parts C and D by December 31, 2010. Improper payments—which largely result from billing mistakes, claims processing errors, and provision of unnecessary services—were estimated to amount to approximately $24.1 billion in 2009.[25] RACs are responsible for reducing Medicare's improper payment rates by identifying underpayments and overpayments made to providers, recovering overpayments, and working with providers to prevent future improper payments. RACs are paid a contingency fee based on a percentage of the overpayments they recover from Medicare providers and suppliers.

Medicare's quality assurance activities are handled by state Survey Agencies and Quality Improvement Organizations (QIOs), which operate in all states, the District of Columbia, Puerto Rico, and the U.S. Virgin Islands. State survey agencies are responsible for inspecting Medicare provider facilities (i.e., nursing homes, home health agencies, and hospitals) to ensure they are in compliance with federal safety and quality standards referred to as Conditions of Participation. QIOs monitor the quality of care delivered to Medicare beneficiaries and educate providers on the latest quality improvement techniques.

PPACA requires the Secretary, no later than January 1, 2011, to establish within CMS a Center for Medicare and Medicaid Innovation (CMI). The purpose of CMI is to test and evaluate innovative payment and service delivery models to reduce program expenditures under Medicare, Medicaid, and CHIP while preserving or enhancing the quality of care furnished under these programs. In selecting the models, the Secretary is required to give preference to those that improve the coordination, quality, and efficiency of health care services.

Financing

Medicare's financial operations are accounted for through two trust funds, the Hospital Insurance (HI) trust fund for Part A and the Supplementary Medical Insurance (SMI) trust fund for Part B, which are maintained by the Department of the Treasury. The HI and SMI trust funds are overseen by a board of trustees that makes annual reports to Congress. HI is primarily funded by payroll taxes, while SMI is funded through general revenue transfers and premiums.

The trust funds are an accounting mechanism; there is no actual transfer of money into and out of a fund. Income to the trust funds is credited to the fund in the form of interest-bearing government securities. Expenditures for services and administrative costs are recorded against the fund. The securities represent obligations that the government has issued to itself. As long as the trust fund has a balance, the Treasury Department is authorized to make payments for it from the U.S. Treasury.

PPACA established a new 15-member Independent Payment Advisory Board that will, beginning in 2014, make recommendations to reduce Medicare spending in years when Medicare costs are projected to exceed a target growth rate. The board's proposals will take effect unless Congress passes an alternative measure that achieves the same level of savings. The board is prohibited from making proposals that ration care, raise taxes, increase Part B premiums, or change Medicare benefit, eligibility, or cost-sharing standards.

Part A Financing

The primary source of funding for Part A is payroll taxes paid by employees and employers.[26] Each pays a tax of 1.45% on the employee's earnings; the self-employed pay 2.9%. Beginning in 2013, some higher-income employees will pay higher payroll taxes and pay taxes on net investment income. Unlike Social Security, there is no upper limit on earnings subject to the tax. Other sources of income include (1) interest on federal securities held by the trust fund, (2) a portion of federal income taxes that individuals pay on their social security benefits, (3) premiums paid by voluntary enrollees who are not automatically entitled to Medicare Part A, (4) transfers from states, and (5) other revenues. Income for Part A is credited to the HI trust fund. Part A expenditures for 2009 are estimated to reach approximately $246 billion.[27]

In 2008, Part A expenditures began to exceed payroll tax income; and, in 2009, the Medicare trustees estimated that the Part A fund would become insolvent by 2017. Subsequent to the enactment of health reform legislation, the Office of the Actuary of CMS estimated that changes made by PPACA to reduce program spending and increase Part A revenues would extend the solvency of the HI trust fund for another 12 years—until 2029.[28]

Part B Financing

Medicare Part B is financed mostly from federal general revenues, with beneficiaries paying premiums equal to 25% of estimated program costs for the aged. (The disabled pay the same premium as the aged.) Income for Part B is credited to the SMI trust fund. General revenue spending for Part B in 2009 is estimated to reach about $164 billion.[29]

The 2010 monthly premium is $96.40 for most established Medicare beneficiaries who voluntarily enroll in Part B.[30] Individuals receiving Social Security benefits have their Part B premium payments automatically deducted from their Social Security benefit checks. An individual's Social Security check cannot go down from one year to the next as a result of the annual Part B premium increase (except in the case of higher-income individuals subject to income-related premiums).

Since 2007, higher-income enrollees pay higher premiums. As a result of PPACA, from 2009 through 2019, individuals whose modified adjusted gross income (AGI) exceeds $85,000 and each member of a couple filing jointly whose modified AGI exceeds $170,000 is subject to higher premium amounts. These higher-income premiums range from 35% to 80% of the value of Part B, affecting about 5% of enrollees in 2009.[31]

Part C Financing

Payments for spending under the Medicare Advantage program are made in appropriate portions from the HI and SMI trust funds. There is no separate trust fund for Part C.

Part D Financing

Medicare Part D is financed through a combination of beneficiary premiums and federal general revenues. In addition, certain transfers are made from the states. These transfers, referred to as "clawback payments," represent a portion of the amounts states could otherwise have been expected to pay for drugs under Medicaid if drug coverage for the dual eligible population had not been transferred to Part D. Part D revenues are credited to a separate Part D account within the SMI trust fund. In 2009, general revenue spending for Part D is estimated to be $49 billion.32

Beneficiaries pay different premiums depending on the plan they have selected (and whether they are entitled to low-income premium subsidies). On average, beneficiary premiums account for 25.5% of expected total Part D costs for basic coverage. Part D premium payments may be automatically deducted from Social Security benefit checks, paid directly to the PDP sponsor or MA-PD organization, or made through an electronic funds transfer.

Additional Insurance Coverage

While Medicare provides broad protection against the costs of many, primarily acute care, services, the program does not cover all services that may be used by its aged and disabled beneficiaries. Medicare does not cover eyeglasses, hearing aids, dentures, or most long-term care services. Further, unlike most private insurance polices, it does not include an annual "catastrophic" cap on out-of-pocket spending on cost-sharing charges for services covered under Parts A and B (except for persons enrolled in regional PPOs under MMA).

Most Medicare beneficiaries have some coverage in addition to Medicare. The following are the main sources of additional coverage for Medicare enrollees.

- Medicare Advantage. Many MA plans offer services in addition to those covered under original Medicare and may also have a catastrophic cap.[33]
- Employer Coverage. Coverage may be provided through a current or former employer. In recent years, a number of employers have cut back on the scope of retiree coverage. Some have dropped such coverage entirely, particularly for future retirees. As noted earlier, the MMA attempted to stem this trend, at least for prescription drug coverage, by offering subsidies to employers who offer drug coverage, at least as good as that available under Part D.
- Medigap. Individual insurance policies that supplement Medicare are referred to as Medigap policies. Beneficiaries with Medigap insurance typically have coverage for a portion of Medicare's deductibles and coinsurance; they may also have coverage for some items and services not covered by Medicare. Individuals generally select one of the standardized plans, though not all plans are offered in all states.
- Medicaid. Certain low-income Medicare beneficiaries also may be eligible for full or partial benefits under their state's Medicaid program. Individuals eligible for both Medicare and Medicaid are referred to as dual eligibles. The lowest- income dual eligibles qualify for full Medicaid benefits, so that the majority of their health care

expenses are paid by either Medicare or Medicaid; Medicare pays first, with Medicaid picking up most of the remaining costs. In addition to full-benefit dual eligibles, state Medicaid programs pay Medicare premiums and some cost-sharing for other partial dual eligibles, who have higher income than full-benefit dual eligibles but are still considered to have low income.[34]

- Other Public Sources. Individuals may have additional coverage through the Department of Veterans Affairs, or TRICARE for military retirees eligible for Medicare (and enrolled in Part B).

In 2007, close to 90% of beneficiaries had some form of additional coverage. (Some persons may have had more than one type of such coverage.)

Medicare Issues

With the enactment of health care reform legislation earlier this year, the remaining months of the 111th Congress may be spent working on addressing Medicare physician payment issues, identifying and making any necessary technical fixes to the March legislation, and considering extensions of Medicare policies that will expire at the end of 2010 (for example, the exceptions process for therapy caps and bonus payments for ground and air ambulance services in rural areas).

Over the longer term, Congress' focus will include monitoring the implementation and effects of payment and program changes made by the health care reform laws to determine, for instance, whether payment reductions are sustainable and whether delivery models being tested through pilot programs and demonstrations have the potential to slow cost growth in medical care and/or improve the quality of services provided.

Some of the key policy issues and questions Congress will likely face include the following:

- A combination of factors have contributed to the rapid growth in Medicare spending. These include increases in overall medical costs, new and increasing use of technology, increases in the percentage of the population over 65, and longer life spans. How will changes made in recent health care reform legislation affect the growth in Medicare expenditures and the long-term solvency of the Medicare Hospital Insurance (Part A) trust fund? How effective will the Independent Payment Advisory Board created by PPACA be in controlling costs? Will existing financing mechanisms be sufficient to support program spending over the long term?
- Medicare cost-sharing is generally higher than it is under private insurance plans for workers. For example, under Medicare there is no limit on out-of-pocket expenditures, limited nursing home and home care services, and significant co-payments for some services. Consequently, many beneficiaries pay additional premiums for insurance to supplement Medicare (e.g., Medigap). How will the level of beneficiary out-of-pocket expenses be affected by health care reform changes? What is the impact of high out-of-pocket costs and gaps in Medicare coverage on beneficiaries' health and access to care?

- Under health care reform legislation, Medicare is tasked with expanding or developing demonstrations and pilot programs to explore whether the use of accountable care organizations (ACO), bundled payments for care provided to a patient across various settings, reduced payments for preventable hospital readmissions, and value-based purchasing can lead to lower medical costs and/or improved quality of care. How long will it take before results can be demonstrated? What elements are key to successful implementation (for example, adequate number of participating primary care providers, advanced and integrated information systems, legal requirements for establishing ACOs, and adequate financial incentives)? Can these models be successful if only used by Medicare and not by other private or public payers?
- PPACA requires Medicare, through the implementation of a Community-Based Care Transitions Program and an Independence at Home Program, to test whether payment for care coordination can result in quality-of-care improvements for chronically ill individuals and reduce unnecessary hospitalization and acute care expenditures. These programs experiment with different kinds of care coordination—that which is delivered to individuals during their transition from a hospital stay into a post-acute or home care setting, and that which is delivered to persons in their homes by primary care physicians and other interdisciplinary teams of nurses, physician assistants, pharmacists, and other health and social services staff. Will payment for care coordination help improve patient outcomes? Can such coordination help to reduce Medicare costs by avoiding preventable admissions to more expensive care settings, such as hospitals and nursing homes?
- CMS was given significant new authority under PPACA to better coordinate care for individuals eligible for both Medicare and Medicaid. In establishing the Center for Medicare and Medicaid Innovation as well as the Federal Coordinated Health Care Office, Congress provided options that can be used to experiment with new service delivery and payment options for beneficiaries of both Medicare and Medicaid. Will these changes help to maintain and improve quality of care while decreasing medical care costs to both the Medicaid and Medicare programs for these dually eligible beneficiaries? What new approaches or authority might be necessary to ensure that acute and long-term care are integrated, while maintaining or improving quality of care for dual eligible and other chronically ill beneficiaries?
- Under PPACA, certain providers, such as hospitals, skilled nursing facilities (SNFs), and home health agencies (HHAs), face permanent reductions in the annual updates to their Medicare payment rates. How will these providers modify services to become more efficient? Will there be a reduction in access to these services for Medicare beneficiaries? Will Medicare payment reductions for these providers lead to higher prices to other payers? Will these reductions result in some providers leaving Medicare or being unable to remain in business?
- Medicare payments to physicians and other providers under the Medicare physician fee schedule continue to grow at rates that require reductions in the reimbursement rates under current law by the sustainable growth rate (SGR) system. While Congress has passed legislation several times to avert these reductions, the search for a long-term solution or replacement for the update formula continues, while each override becomes more costly. Additionally, the longstanding issue with Medicare's physician

payments and the potential for future reductions has accelerated concern that Medicare beneficiaries will be increasingly unable to access providers. What will the impact be on access to care due to increased demand for health care services as a result of PPACA's Medicaid expansions and the expected growth in the number of insured in the private sector? How will the rates paid on behalf of these new covered groups compare with Medicare rates, and would providers be more willing to provide care to one population over another?

- PPACA changed how the maximum possible payments to MA plans will be calculated by first tying them closer to or below the level of spending in original Medicare and by adjusting them based on plan quality. This may result in payment reductions for many MA plans. How will changes to Medicare Advantage plan payments affect the availability of plans and the types of supplemental benefits and reduced cost-sharing that they offer? Will the payment changes encourage higher plan quality or encourage enrollees to switch to higher quality MA plans?
- PPACA made a number of changes affecting the Medicare Part D prescription drug program, including mandating a 50% manufacturer discount on brand name drugs for enrollees in the coverage gap and a gradual phasing out of the "doughnut hole." How will the phase-out of the doughnut hole affect beneficiaries' out-of-pockets costs and their ability to access needed prescriptions? How many manufacturers will provide 50% discounts for brand name drugs in the coverage gap? Will Medicare cover drugs that are medically needed but whose manufacturers did not enter into an agreement to provide the discount? What will happen to drug prices over time? What will be the impact of the gap closure on total Medicare Part D expenditures?
- Program integrity provisions in PPACA increased resources, added new requirements, enhanced activities to prevent fraud and abuse, and increased uniformity in program integrity activities among Medicare, Medicaid, and the State Children's Health Insurance Program (CHIP). Will these changes be sufficient to deter potentially fraudulent providers from entering the program, while at the same time not being so burdensome as to discourage legitimate providers from participating in Medicare? Will CMS, its contractors, and oversight agencies be better able to prevent improper payments from being paid in the first place and reduce the reliance on the "pay-and-chase" approach? How much savings will be realized from these new authorities and activities; and how can this savings best be measured? Will additional authorities or new approaches be needed?

Acknowledgments

The authors wish to thank Hinda Chaikind, who coordinated and wrote an earlier version of this report.

End Notes

[1] Also known as "customary, prevailing and reasonable charges," this method based physician payments on charges commonly used by physicians in a local community. The payment for a service was the lowest of (1) the physician's billed charge for the service, (2) the physician's customary charge for the service, or (3) the prevailing charge for that service in the community.

[2] ESRD is a stage of kidney impairment that appears to be irreversible and permanent, requiring a regular course of dialysis treatments or a kidney transplantation to maintain life.

[3] For more information, see CRS Report RL3 1966, *Overview of the Medicare Prescription Drug, Improvement, and Modernization Act of 2003.*

[4] For more information, see CRS Report RL34360, *P.L. 110-173: Provisions in the Medicare, Medicaid, and SCHIP Extension Act of 2007.*

[5] For more information, see CRS Report RL34592, *P.L. 110-2 75: The Medicare Improvements for Patients and Providers Act of 2008.*

[6] For more information, see CRS Report R41 196, *Medicare Provisions in the Patient Protection and Affordable Care Act (PPACA): Summary and Timeline.*

[7] Groups of providers and suppliers who work together to manage and coordinate care for Medicare fee-for-service beneficiaries.

[8] For more information, see CRS Report RS22 195, *Social Security Disability Insurance (SSDI) and Medicare: The 24- Month Waiting Period for SSDI Beneficiaries Under Age 65.*

[9] Because there was no Social Security cost-of-living adjustment (COLA) in 2010 due to the economic slowdown, a statutory hold-harmless provision protected established Medicare beneficiaries from Part B premium increases. However, the provision did not apply to certain categories of beneficiaries and some beneficiaries are paying higher Part B premiums in 2010. See CRS Report R40561, *The Effect of No Social Security COLA on Medicare Part B Premiums*, by Jim Hahn and Alison M. Shelton.

[10] Additionally, starting in 2011, MA enrollees will only be permitted to drop out of their MA plans and return to original Medicare during the first 45-day period of each calendar year—they will no longer be allowed to switch to another MA plan as they were able to do previously. MA enrollees will still be able to switch plans during special enrollment periods, such as when an MA enrollee moves outside his or her plan's service area or if an enrollee's MA plan is terminated.

[11] If a Medicare beneficiary enrolls in a Private Fee-for-Service (PFFS) plan that does not provide drug coverage, he or she may enroll in a stand-alone Prescription Drug Plan (PDP). However, enrollees in other types of MA plans who want Part D prescription drug coverage must choose a Medicare Advantage Prescription Drug (MA-PD) plan, which is an MA plan that provides all Medicare required parts A, B, and D benefits. If a Medicare beneficiary enrolls in a local HMO or regional PPO that does not offer drug coverage, he or she does not have the option to enroll in a stand-alone PDP plan.

[12] Hospitals in the state of Maryland are exempt from the IPPS and are paid under a state-specific payment system.

[13] By October 1, 2013, the Secretary will be required to implement budget neutral revisions to the methodology for determining hospice payments for routine home care and other services. These revisions could include adjustments to the per diem payments reflecting differences in resources used during the course of an entire episode of hospice care.

[14] For details, see the Annual Reports of the Board of Trustees of the Federal Hospital Insurance and Federal Supplementary Medical Insurance Trust Funds.

[15] This "mental health parity" was introduced in MIPPA (P.L. 110-275).

[16] For details, see CRS Report R40907, *Medicare Physician Payment Updates and the Sustainable Growth Rate (SGR) System*, by Jim Hahn.

[17] For details, see CRS Report R41196, *Medicare Provisions in the Patient Protection and Affordable Care Act (PPACA): Summary and Timeline.*

[18] See General Accounting Office (GAO) report, "Medicare Payments for Oxygen," May 15, 1997, GAO-97-120R; HHS Office of the Inspector General report, "Medicare Home Oxygen Equipment: Cost and Servicing," September 2006, OEI-09-04-00420.

[19] For more information, see CRS Report R4121 1, *Medicare Durable Medical Equipment: The Competitive Bidding Program.*

[20] Biologics are generally derived from living organisms rather than inorganic chemical compounds.

[21] Additionally, starting in 2006, rural sole community hospitals (SCHs) receive an additional 7.1% in Medicare payments. Special payment protections apply to cancer hospitals, children's hospitals, small rural hospitals (that are not SCHs) with 100 or fewer beds, and SCHs.

[22] New, office-based procedures are services that are performed in physician offices at least 50% of the time. Payment is set at the lower of the ASC rate or the practice expense portion of the physician fee schedule payment rate.

[23] For additional information, see CRS Report R41 196, *Medicare Provisions in the Patient Protection and Affordable Care Act (PPACA): Summary and Timeline*.

[24] For more information on Medicare contractors and Medicare fraud and abuse, see CRS Report RL34217, *Medicare Program Integrity: Activities to Protect Medicare from Payment Errors, Fraud, and Abuse*.

[25] Total improper payments include both overpayments and underpayments. In FY2009, overpayments were estimated to be $23 billion and underpayments $1.1 billion. For more information, see the *Executive Summary, Improper Medicare FFS Payments Report*, November 2009, available at http://www.cms.gov/CERT/ Downloads/ CERT_Report.pdf.

[26] For more information on the Part A financing, see CRS Report RS20 173, *Medicare: Financing the Part A Hospital Insurance Program* and CRS Report RS20946, *Medicare: History of Part A Trust Fund Insolvency Projections*.

[27] 2009 Annual Report of the Boards of Trustees of the Federal Hospital Insurance and Federal Supplementary Medical Insurance Trust Funds, Table III.B4, p. 52, http://www.cms.hhs.gov/reportstrustfunds/.

[28] Memorandum from Solomon M. Mussey, "Estimated Effects of the 'Patient Protection and Affordable Care Act,' as Amended, on the Year of Exhaustion for the Part A Trust Fund, Part B Premiums, and Part A and Part B Coinsurance Amounts," April 22, 2010, http://www.cms.gov/ActuarialStudies/Downloads/PPACA_ Medicare_2010-04-22.pdf.

[29] 2009 Annual Report of the Boards of Trustees of the Federal Hospital Insurance and Federal Supplementary Medical Insurance Trust Funds, Table III.C8, p. 96, http://www.cms.hhs.gov/reportstrustfunds/.

[30] For more information, see CRS Report R40561, *The Effect of No Social Security COLA on Medicare Part B Premiums*.

[31] The higher monthly premium amounts for 2010 are based on 2008 income levels and are (1) $ 154.70—for single beneficiaries with income $85,001-$107,000 or for each member of a couple filing jointly with income $170,001- $214,000; (2) $221.00—for single beneficiaries with income $107,001-$160,000 or for each member of a couple filing jointly with income $214,001-$320,000; (3) $287.30—for single beneficiaries with incomes $160,001-$214,000 and each member of a couple filing jointly with income $320,001-$428,000; and (4) $353.60—for single beneficiaries with incomes greater than $214,000 and each member of a couple filing jointly income above $428,000. The 2010 income thresholds are the same as for 2009, and PPACA freezes these thresholds through 2019 at 2010 levels.

[32] 2009 Annual Report of the Boards of Trustees of the Federal Hospital Insurance and Federal Supplementary Medical Insurance Trust Funds, Table III.C19, p.120, http://www.cms.hhs.gov/reportstrustfunds/.

[33] In 2010, Regional MA plans are required to have a catastrophic cap on out-of-pocket (OOP) spending, while some local MA plans also include a cap. Starting in 2011, all MA plans will be required to include a maximum OOP limit determined by CMS.

[34] In addition to individuals eligible for full Medicaid benefits, other low-income Medicare beneficiaries are entitled to limited benefits under the Medicare Savings Program (MSP). MSP includes three benefit categories each with different benefit levels: (1) Qualified Medicare Beneficiaries (QMBs), (2) Specified Low-Income Beneficiaries (SLMB), and (3) Qualified Individuals (QIs). For QMBs, state Medicaid programs pay Medicare Part B premiums and Medicare cost- sharing (deductibles and co-payments) when beneficiaries' incomes are under 100% of the federal poverty level (FPL). For SLMBs, state Medicaid programs pay Part B premiums when beneficiaries' incomes are between 100% and 120% of the FPL. For QIs, Medicaid pays premiums when beneficiaries' incomes are between 120% and 135% of poverty. To be eligible for MSP, Medicare beneficiaries must also meet Medicaid's other eligibility requirements (e.g., meet citizenship or legal residency requirements).

Index

X